THE GASTROINTESTINAL TRACT

INTERNATIONAL ACADEMY OF PATHOLOGY

MONOGRAPHS IN PATHOLOGY

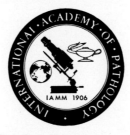

SERIES EDITOR, Murray R. Abell, M.D.

Professor, Department of Pathology,
University of Michigan Medical School, Ann Arbor, Michigan

No. 1. The Lymphocyte and Lymphocytic Tissue
JOHN W. REBUCK *and* ROBERT E. STOWELL, *Editors*
No. 2. The Adrenal Cortex
HENRY D. MOON *and* ROBERT E. STOWELL, *Editors*
No. 3. The Ovary
HUGH G. GRADY *and* DAVID E. SMITH, *Editors*
No. 4. The Peripheral Blood Vessels
J. LOWELL ORBISON *and* DAVID E. SMITH, *Editors*
No. 5. The Thyroid
J. BEACH HAZARD *and* DAVID E. SMITH, *Editors*
No. 6. The Kidney
F. K. MOSTOFI *and* DAVID E. SMITH, *Editors*
No. 7. The Connective Tissue
BERNARD M. WAGNER *and* DAVID E. SMITH, *Editors*
No. 8. The Lung
AVERILL A. LIEBOW *and* DAVID E. SMITH, *Editors*
No. 9. The Brain
ORVILLE T. BAILEY *and* DAVID E. SMITH, *Editors*
No. 10. The Skin
ELSON B. HELWIG *and* F. K. MOSTOFI, *Editors*
No. 11. The Platelet
K. M. BRINKHOUS, R. W. SHERMER, *and* F. K. MOSTOFI, *Editors*
No. 12. The Striated Muscle
CARL M. PEARSON *and* F. K. MOSTOFI, *Editors*
No. 13. The Liver
EDWARD A. GALL *and* F. K. MOSTOFI, *Editors*
No. 14. The Uterus
HENRY J. NORRIS, ARTHUR T. HERTIG *and* MURRAY R. ABELL, *Editors*
No. 15. The Heart
JESSE E. EDWARDS, MAURICE LEV, *and* MURRAY R. ABELL, *Editors*
No. 16. The Reticuloendothelial System
JOHN W. REBUCK, COSTAN W. BERARD, *and* MURRAY R. ABELL, *Editors*
No. 17. Bones and Joints
LAUREN V. ACKERMAN, HARLAN J. SPJUT, *and* MURRAY R. ABELL, *Editors*
No. 18. The Gastrointestinal Tract
JOHN H. YARDLEY, BASIL C. MORSON *and* MURRAY R. ABELL, *Editors*
Succeeding Volumes to Be Announced

INTERNATIONAL ACADEMY OF PATHOLOGY MONOGRAPH

THE GASTROINTESTINAL TRACT

by 21 authors

EDITED BY **JOHN H. YARDLEY, M.D.**

Department of Pathology, The Johns Hopkins University,
Baltimore, Maryland

BASIL C. MORSON, D.M., F.R.C.Path.

Department of Pathology, St. Mark's Hospital, London, England

AND MURRAY R. ABELL, M.D.

Department of Pathology
University of Michigan, Medical School, Ann Arbor, Michigan

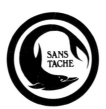

The Williams & Wilkins Company
Baltimore, 1977

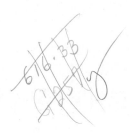

Library of Congress Cataloging in Publication Data
Main entry under title:

The Gastrointestinal Tract.

(Monographs in pathology; no. 18)
1. Intestines – Cancer. 2. Stomach – Cancer. 3. Intestines – Diseases. 4. Stomach – Diseases. I. Yardley, John H. II. Morson, B. C. III. Abell, Murray R. IV. Series: International Academy of Pathology. Monographs in pathology; no. 18. [DNLM: 1. Gastrointestinal diseases. 2. Gastrointestinal neoplasms. W1 M0568H no. 18 / WI149 G257]
RC280.I8G37   616.3'3   76-30330 683-09317-7

COMPOSED AND PRINTED AT
WAVERLY PRESS, INC.
Mt. Royal and Guilford Aves.
Baltimore, MD. 21202, U.S.A.

Contents

Contributing Authors

NEIL R. BLACKLOW, M.D.
  Chief, Section of Infectious Diseases, University of Massachusetts, Medical Center, Worcester, Massachusetts

MARK DONOWITZ, M.D.
  Department of Gastroenterology, Walter Reed Army Institute of Research, Washington, D.C.

WILHELM G. DOOS, M.D.
  Associate Pathologist, Mallory Institute of Pathology, Boston City Hospital, Boston, Massachusetts

S. B. FORMAL, PH.D.
  Chief, Department of Applied Immunology, Division of Communicable Disease and Immunology, Walter Reed Army Institute of Research, Walter Reed Army Medical Center, Washington, D.C.

P. GEMSKI, JR., PH.D.
  Assistant Chief, Department of Applied Immunology, Division of Communicable Disease and Immunology, Walter Reed Army Institute of Research, Walter Reed Army Medical Center, Washington, D.C.

LEONARD S. GOTTLIEB, M.D., M.P.H.
  Director, Mallory Institute of Pathology, Boston City Hospital, Boston, Massachusetts

M. J. HILL, PH.D., M.R.C.Path.
  Director, Bacterial Metabolism Research Laboratory, Central Public Health Laboratory, London, England

NATHAN LANE, M.D.
  Division of Surgical Pathology, Columbia University, College of Physicians and Surgeons, New York, New York

BENJAMIN B. LURIE, M.D.
  Research Associate (Pathology), Gastrointestinal Research Laboratory, Mallory Institute of Pathology, Boston City Hospital, Boston, Massachusetts

VINCENT J. McGOVERN, M.D.
  Director, Fairfax Institute of Pathology, Royal Prince Alfred Hospital, Camperdown, Australia

BASIL C. MORSON, D.M., F.R.C.Path.
  Department of Pathology, St. Mark's Hospital, London, England

SI-CHUN MING, M.D.
> *Department of Pathology, Temple University, School of Medicine, Philadelphia, Pennsylvania*

H. THOMAS NORRIS, M.D.
> *Director, Hospital Pathology, University of Washington, School of Medicine, Seattle, Washington*

A. G. E. PEARSE, M.D., F.R.C. Path.
> *Royal Postgraduate Medical School, London, England*

ASHLEY B. PRICE, M.R.C. Path.
> *Histopathology Department, Northwick Park Hospital and Clinical Research Centre, Harrow, Middlesex, England*

ROMULO PRUDENTE, M.D.
> *Research Assistant (Pathology), Gastrointestinal Research Laboratory, Mallory Institute of Pathology, Boston City Hospital, Boston, Massachusetts*

ROBERT H. RIDDELL, M.D.
> *Department of Pathology, The University of Chicago, Chicago, Illinois*

DAVID S. SCHREIBER, M.D.
> *Gastroenterology Division, Peter Bent Brigham Hospital, Boston, Massachusetts*

JERRY S. TRIER, M.D.
> *Director, Gastroenterology Division, Peter Bent Brigham Hospital, Boston, Massachusetts*

JOHN H. YARDLEY, M.D.
> *The Johns Hopkins University, Department of Pathology, Baltimore, Maryland*

NORMAN ZAMCHECK, M.D.
> *Chief, Gastrointestinal Research Laboratory, Mallory Institute of Pathology, Boston City Hospital, Boston, Massachusetts*

Foreword

This Monograph is the 18th in the series of yearly Monographs in Pathology initiated by the International Academy of Pathology in 1959. It is the first in the series to deal with diseases of the gastrointestinal system. Each monograph in the series represents a compilation of lectures and illustrative materials born of the annual Long Course sponsored by the Council of the United States-Canadian Division of the Academy. The Long Courses and their progeny, the monographs, comprise a major and vital facet of the Academy's educational program and contribute greatly to the realization of its goal to assemble for its membership educational material of the finest scientific quality. "Inflammatory and Neoplastic Diseases of the Gastrointestinal Tract" comprised the Long Course at the 65th Annual Meeting of the United States-Canadian Division of the International Academy of Pathology in Boston on the 25th of March, 1976. The offspring, this monograph, forms a permanent and readily accessible record of that course.

The Directors of the Long Course for 1976, Dr. John H. Yardley and Dr. Basil C. Morson, assembled an impressive faculty of scientists and their presentations in this monograph comprise a rich deposit of knowledge for use by all who have an interest in or seek further understanding of gastrointestinal diseases. Each chapter represents a distillate of much important investigative work and contributes greatly to our current understanding of gastrointestinal disease. The monograph is a monument to each investigator's industry and accomplishments.

The Council and the Executive Committee of the United States-Canadian Division of the Academy express their sincere appreciation to Dr. Yardley and Dr. Morson and to their distinguished faculty who contributed their time and knowledge to the preparation of this monograph and to the publishers, The Williams & Wilkins Company, for their encouragment and support.

M. R. ABELL, M.D., PH.D.
Series Editor

Preface

This monograph comprises, in expanded form, presentations made at the Long Course on Inflammatory and Neoplastic Disease of the Gastrointestinal Tract held during the annual meeting of the International Academy of Pathology, United States-Canadian Division, in Boston, Massachusetts on March 25, 1976.

Editors of monographs in this series customarily note that their discipline has recently made tremendous strides and that many new and exciting subjects were available for discussion. Gastrointestinal pathology provides every reason to continue this tradition. For, like other sciences, during the past few years the field of gastroenterology has been revolutionized by successful application of many modern investigative and diagnostic tools. Accompanying this general advance, and, indeed, often at its forefront, has been progress in recognizing and understanding the pathological processes that accompany gastrointestinal disease. Development of ingenious devices such as peroral biopsy capsules and fiberscopes has, of course, greatly aided these advances.

It was manifestly impossible to cover all forms of gastrointestinal disease in a one-day conference. We decided, therefore, to concentrate on two areas, inflammatory and neoplastic diseases, since advances in disease classification, in disease mechanisms, and in development of new diagnostic techniques have been especially numerous in both areas.

While it was not possible to be exhaustive even over the relatively small subject areas of inflammatory and neoplastic disease, we have attempted to assemble a balanced collection of presentations on these subjects. At the same time, a central purpose was to concentrate on topics that would bear on the day-to-day activities of the diagnostic histopathologist. Thus, newer approaches to classifying and to recognizing various forms of inflammatory disease and tumors are described along with discussions of special diagnostic procedures like the CEA test. In addition, such etiologic and pathogenetic factors as ischemia, bacterial and viral agents in inflammatory bowel disease are considered. For colonic cancer, studies on adenomas and effects of the intralumenal environment are discussed.

We wish to express our gratitude to each of the authors for contributing their time, energy and knowledge to this symposium. We also thank the International Academy of Pathology for the opportunity to organize the Long Course and this monograph.

JOHN H. YARDLEY, M.D.
BASIL C. MORSON, D.M., F.R.C.Path.

Chapter 1

Difficulties in the Differential Diagnosis of Ulcerative Colitis and Crohn's Disease

ASHLEY B. PRICE

Two problems face the histopathologist: 1) the separation of Crohn's disease and ulcerative colitis from other types of inflammatory bowel disease, and 2) the separation of colonic Crohn's disease and ulcerative colitis from each other.

The differential diagnosis of nonspecific inflammatory bowel disease is shown in Figure 1. There are many articles on this subject[12, 16] and some of the conditions listed will be dealt with elsewhere in this monograph. Here attention is focused on the second problem, the separation of Crohn's disease of the colon from ulcerative colitis. In particular, the problem of the atypical case that is difficult to classify is considered.[4, 10]

The colon has a limited range of response to disease so that many of the histopathologic features of Crohn's disease and ulcerative colitis are shared. While the etiologies remain unknown the distinguishing characteristics must necessarily be subjective and are often ill-defined. For example, how precisely can one distinguish a fissure from undermining ulceration, or define the depth of inflammation in ulcerative colitis? No one feature is invariably present in one disease and considerable diversity exists within one specimen. The effects of treatment, rate of onset of the disease, age, and patient individuality on the pathology are also poorly understood. Indeed, it is still debated whether Crohn's disease and ulcerative colitis are two distinct diseases or opposite ends of the spectrum of one disease. A diagnostic problem will continue to exist until the etiologies are discovered or improved diagnostic criteria are found.

ULCERATIVE COLITIS AND CROHN'S DISEASE (THE TYPICAL CASE)

Despite these difficulties a distinction between colonic Crohn's disease and ulcerative colitis can be confidently made in up to 90% of cases, using certain clinical, radiologic, and histopathologic criteria.[11] The major pathologic distinguishing features, clearly described by Lockhart-Mummery and Morson,[11] are well known. When they are all present the differentiation of the two diseases is straightforward. Ulcerative colitis is a disease confined to the large bowel that commences in the rectum and spreads proximally. It is primarily a mucosal disease characterized by recurrent bouts of inflammation, ulceration, and regen-

1

Gastrointestinal Tract

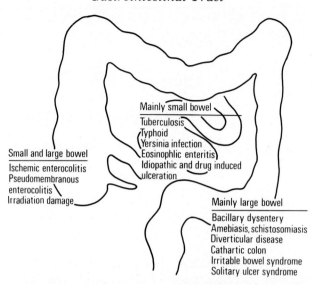

Mainly small bowel
Tuberculosis
Typhoid
Yersinia infection
Eosinophlic enteritis
Idiopathic and drug induced
ulceration

Small and large bowel
Ischemic enterocolitis
Pseudomembranous
enterocolitis
Irradiation damage

Mainly large bowel
Bacillary dysentery
Amebiasis, schistosomiasis
Diverticular disease
Cathartic colon
Irritable bowel syndrome
Solitary ulcer syndrome

The differential diagnosis of Crohn's disease and ulcerative colitis

FIG. 1. Differential diagnosis of Crohn's disease and ulcerative colitis. (Reproduced from: A. B. Price and B. C. Morson: *Human Pathology 6:* 7–29, 1975.)

eration that lead eventually to mucosal atrophy, and in certain cases, to carcinoma. Mucosal glandular irregularity and goblet cell depletion are prominent in the established case. The bowel wall only becomes involved in the acute, severe phase. Crohn's disease, on the other hand, affects the whole wall and is a disease of both small and large intestine. It has a tendency to involve the right side of the colon more than the left. Skip lesions, fistulae, and strictures are characteristic. Histologically fissuring ulceration, sarcoid-like granulomas, and transmural inflammation with an aggregated pattern are typical. A regular mucosa containing normal goblet cells in the presence of an inflammatory infiltrate contrasts with that seen in ulcerative colitis. Precancerous changes have not been described.

Since these descriptions of colonic Crohn's disease and ulcerative colitis there have been many attempts to be more selective and to separate features of major diagnostic importance. The technique of discriminant analysis[7] has shown the significance of the goblet cell population, and morphometry[20] has also been used to try to improve diagnostic accuracy. Recently this method has demonstrated that the uninvolved "normal rectum" in Crohn's disease contains increased numbers of plasma cells and the lamina propria has an increased volume.[5] Cook and Dixon[2] analysed over 90 attributes in nonspecific inflammatory bowel disease before concluding that in only a select few was there accurate observer agreement, and these were the most helpful in the differential diagnosis. The sarcoid-like granuloma is still perhaps the only absolute distinguishing feature. Figure 2 shows those features generally accepted as having the best positive discriminating value.[2, 9] The less specific features that are more common in one condition than the other, such as lymphangiectasia and neuronal hyperplasia, add confidence to what must be a final cumulative diagnosis.

COLONIC CROHN'S DISEASE

A discontinuous disease pattern
Macroscopic deep fissures and confluent linear ulceration
Microscopic fissuring ulceration
Sarcoid-like granulomas
Ulcerating lymphoid follicles
A regular mucosal glandular pattern in the presence of inflammatory cell infiltration
A well maintained goblet cell population
Transmural inflammation with an aggregated pattern
Submucosal fibrosis

ULCERATIVE COLITIS

Macroscopically a healed granular mucosa spreading proximally in continuity with rectal disease
An absence of fissures
A continuous pattern of inflammation confined to the mucosa
An irregular glandular pattern
Goblet cell depletion

Fig. 2. Attributes with positive discriminating value in nonspecific inflammatory bowel disease.

COLITIS UNCLASSIFIED (THE PROBLEM CASE)

To focus on the problems of distinguishing colonic Crohn's disease from ulcerative colitis, those cases that had caused diagnostic difficulty, seen at St. Mark's Hospital between 1960 and 1973, were reviewed. There were 30 such cases of "colitis unclassified" taken from over 300 colectomies for nonspecific inflammatory bowel disease carried out during this period. This figure of 10% for colitis unclassified is similar to that in other series.[2, 4, 7] A case was indexed colitis unclassified when no *confident* histopathologic diagnosis could be made on the colectomy or proctocolectomy specimen at the time of surgery. Clinical details were not considered. In all but 6 cases a tentative opinion was given on which form of disease they most resembled. This was to facilitate the future management of the patient.

Colitis unclassified must not be regarded as a definitive diagnosis, though the cases do show a recognizable pattern. It is an expression of doubt, a statement that at one point in time, when surgery was performed, the findings were equivocal. In such circumstances a dynamic view of the disease process may lead to a confident diagnosis when preoperative or follow-up biopsies are assessed.

According to the degree of doubt three diagnostic terms were employed: 1) Colitis unclassified (6 cases), 2) Colitis unclassified — probably/possibly Crohn's disease (12 cases), 3) Colitis unclassified — probably/possibly ulcerative colitis (12 cases). At the same time operation-matched specimens from 25 cases of established ulcerative colitis and 21 cases of confidently diagnosed Crohn's disease were examined.

Two other studies have considered in detail the atypical cases of nonspecific inflammatory bowel disease. The categories here correspond to groups B and C in the report by Glotzer *et al.*[4] and to groups 2 and 3 in the paper by Lewin and Swales.[10] Common to all groups were features which were atypical for ulcerative colitis, yet lacked enough cumulative characteristics for a confident diagnosis of Crohn's disease.

Certain recurring histopathologic features, discussed below, were responsible for the diagnostic doubt in these 30 cases, and figures quoted later suggest that these are the expressions of a common pattern present during an acute and severe attack of either disease.

MACROSCOPIC FEATURES

No unified macroscopic picture was present, the fundamental difficulty being the interpretation of a total severe colitis (23 cases). Apart from this two other patterns were noted. In one, rectal sparing, perhaps accentuated by vigorous treatment with preoperative steroid enemas, gave a false impression of segmental disease (7 cases) (Fig. 3). This pattern was also noted by Schachter, Goldstein, Rappaport, Fennessy, and Kirsner.[19] In the second, variation in the intensity of the disease in different parts of the colon gave an erroneous impression of skip lesions (6 cases) (Fig. 4). Both of these patterns suggested a macroscopic diagnosis of Crohn's disease and yet half the cases in both groups were thought subsequently at microscopy to be more like ulcerative colitis.

FISSURING ULCERATION

A form of fissuring ulceration was seen in 18 of the 30 cases. In 6 of these, other criteria favored a tentative diagnosis of ulcerative colitis. Schachter *et al.*[19] found fissures in 18 of 79 cases that otherwise resembled ulcerative colitis. The fissure is believed to be strongly suggestive of Crohn's disease but occurs in

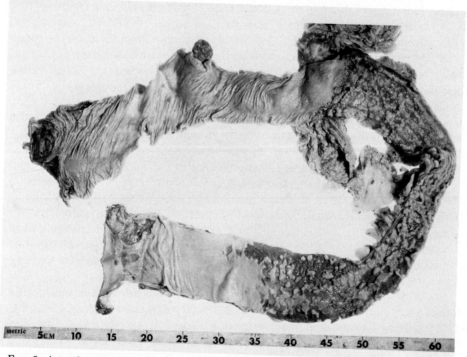

FIG. 3. A total proctocolectomy specimen showing rectal sparing. A misleading macroscopic feature in the acute phase of inflammatory bowel disease. This case showed other features more in favor of a diagnosis of ulcerative colitis.

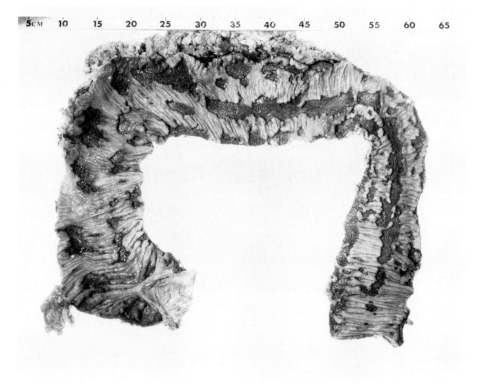

Fig. 4. The variation in intensity of the disease during the acute phase can produce a picture resembling the skip-lesions of typical Crohn's disease. This case showed the typical histology of ulcerative colitis in the subsequent proctectomy.

only 30% of cases,[6] and is often difficult to distinguish from undermining ulceration.

Not enough attention has been drawn to the differences between fissuring in acute disease, the form seen here, and the fissure of classical Crohn's disease. The latter originates in a surface ulcer and runs to a variable depth through the bowel wall often branching in a serpiginous fashion. The fissures are lined by inflammatory cells but mucosa and healthy muscle can commonly be seen nearby (Fig. 5). They are usually single. The fissures in this series, whether cases of doubtful Crohn's disease or ulcerative colitis, occurred in areas of severe ulceration and were often multiple. They took the form of V-shaped clefts or cracks in the muscle which were lined by inflammatory cells (Figs. 6 and 7). The characteristic myocytolysis and capillary engorgement of incipient dilatation were frequently present in the adjacent muscle. This form of fissure is therefore of no discriminative value. It is most misleading when single or seen in an area where extensive mucosal stripping has not yet occurred (Fig. 8).

THE MUCOSAL GLANDULAR PATTERN AND GOBLET CELL POPU-LATION

The regular epithelial pattern of typical Crohn's disease with a preserved goblet cell population, in the presence of severe inflammation contrasts with the

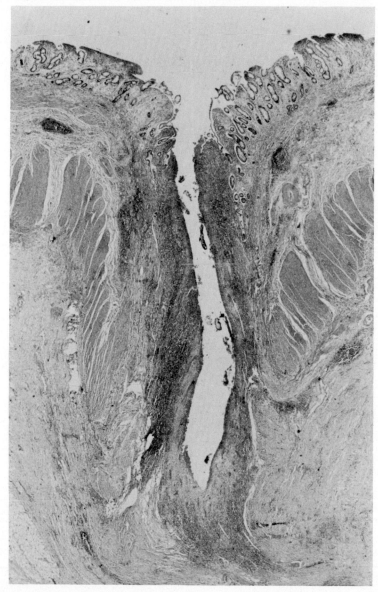

FIG. 5. The typical fissure of Crohn's disease, for comparison with Figures 6–8. Hematoxylin and eosin × 22.5.

mucin depleted, irregular, branched, and atrophic glandular pattern of chronic ulcerative colitis. In these 30 cases these parameters were obscured or modified by extensive ulceration and stripping of the mucosa. Where islands of mucosa remained, the inflammation was surprisingly mild and the epithelium regular with a well maintained goblet cell population (Figs. 8 and 9). This feature favors Crohn's disease. However, it predominated in 4 of the 12 cases in which, because of certain other features, ulcerative colitis was suggested as the provisional diagnosis. It seems probable that extensive and sudden mucosal ulceration

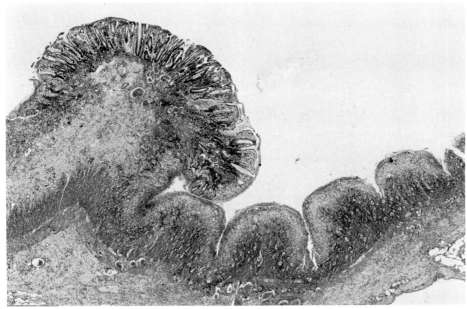

FIG. 6. Acute dilatation (toxic megacolon). The final stage of the acute phase of inflammatory bowel disease. Multiple acute clefts are seen and intense transmural vascular engorgement. The surviving mucosal island is still "relatively" free from inflammation. This case was proven to be ulcerative colitis, showing the typical histology at subsequent proctectomy. Hematoxylin and eosin × 22.

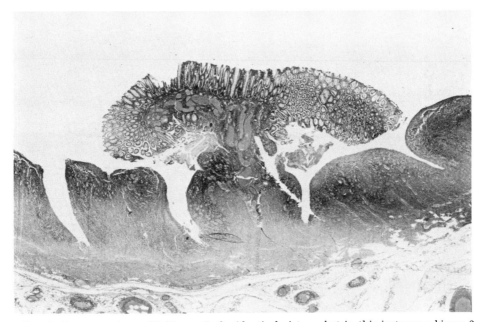

FIG. 7. For comparison with Figure 6, the identical picture, but in this instance a biopsy 2 years earlier had shown unequivocal Crohn's disease, including granulomas. In established acute dilatation the histopathologic overlap between ulcerative colitis and Crohn's disease can be complete. Hematoxylin and eosin × 16.

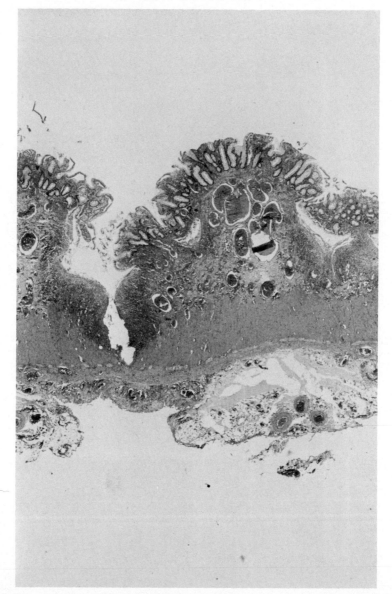

FIG. 8. The acute phase of inflammatory bowel disease. The mucosa still shows a well maintained goblet cell population with little inflammatory infiltration and glandular distortion. An
acute fissure is also seen. This was a case in which no tentative diagnosis could be offered. The
clinical diagnosis was also equivocal. Hematoxylin and eosin × 22.5.

might strip the most diseased regions first, leaving behind the less damaged
mucosal islands. Pseudopolyps, signposts of previous severe ulceration seen in
many more typical cases of nonspecific inflammatory bowel disease, are frequently covered by normal mucosa. This, along with the macroscopic appearance seen in Figure 4, support such a concept. The intensive steroid therapy
received by most of these severely ill patients may also have an effect resulting

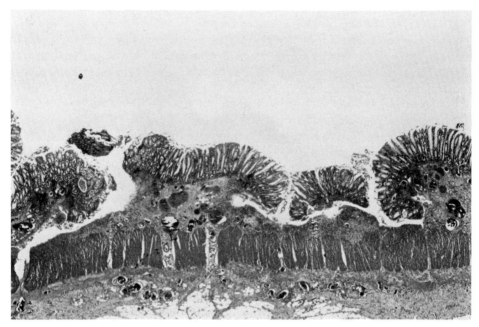

FIG. 9. The developing acute phase of inflammatory bowel disease. Severe ulceration and mucosal stripping has commenced. The surviving mucosa is, however, still regular, and the mucosal inflammation is mild despite cumulative evidence suggesting a diagnosis of "probable" ulcerative colitis. Hematoxylin and eosin × 16.

in the preservation of the goblet cell population.[19] Thus areas showing a regular glandular pattern with a preserved goblet cell population should be interpreted with caution in the severe acute case.

THE INFLAMMATORY INFILTRATE

Twenty-eight of the 30 cases showed areas of transmural inflammation associated with severe ulceration. A dense band of lymphocytes and plasma cells frequently formed the floor of these ulcers. The acceptable limit on the depth of inflammation is a continual problem in ulcerative colitis. In chronic cases it is confined to the mucosa and upper submucosa, but as the degree of ulceration and activity of the disease increase so does the extent of the inflammation.

In only 2 cases was an aggregated pattern of lymphocytes seen. The pattern was a constant feature in all of the control cases of Crohn's disease. McGovern and Goulston[13] emphasize the importance of the aggregated inflammatory pattern in Crohn's disease, and Cook and Dixon[2] found it to be a reliable feature. It has most significance when seen in the muscularis propria and serosa. Aggregates in the submucosa are less significant. In the rectum, where there is already a concentration of lymphoid elements, extra care in interpretation is needed. The reason for the virtual absence of lymphoid aggregates in these cases is not clear. If they were the consequence of a chronic inflammatory reaction, or an immunologic response, one might expect a reduced incidence in a series of severe and mainly acute cases.

THE SARCOID-LIKE GRANULOMA

No granulomas were present in any of the surgical specimens. In each case an average of 11 slides was carefully studied. The granuloma is perhaps the one feature on which histopathologists are prepared to make an absolute distinction between Crohn's disease and ulcerative colitis, but they are present in only 60% of Crohn's cases.[15] The incidence in the control group in this study was similar.

The absence of granulomas might have been chance but if they represent a chronic tissue reaction, as suggested by Whitehead,[21] then, as with lymphoid aggregates, one might again expect a low incidence in this series. At variance with this observation Glass and Baker[3] found granulomas in 50% of cases of Crohn's disease who developed toxic megacolon. An overall incidence in acute disease is difficult to ascertain, for many reports either are without pathology, or the colectomy was performed later in a less acute phase.

TOXIC MEGACOLON, VASCULAR ENGORGEMENT, AND MUSCLE DEGENERATION

Intense transmural vascular congestion and disintegration of muscle is a recognized feature of established toxic megacolon[18] (Figs. 6 and 7). It was present in all 13 cases with radiologically proven dilatation greater than 6 cm. (8 colitis unclassified—possibly ulcerative colitis; 3 colitis unclassified—possibly Crohn's disease; 2 colitis—unclassified—no diagnosis). In addition focal areas with similar changes were seen in 8 of the 17 remaining cases.

The fully established picture of colonic dilatation seen in the 13 cases is the point of maximum overlap in the histopathology of Crohn's disease and ulcerative colitis (Figs. 6 and 7). It is a more frequent complication in ulcerative colitis than in Crohn's disease.[1] The focal changes in 8 cases are an indication of the acute nature of the disease with dilatation being imminent. They are a warning that other atypical features may be present.

GENERAL DISCUSSION

The above observations suggest that in acute and extensive colonic Crohn's disease and ulcerative colitis difficulties in diagnosis are due to two factors. Firstly, fewer of the diagnostic parameters are seen, and secondly, an increase in certain common histopathologic features occurs. A point is reached when on cumulative attributes a confident diagnosis can no longer be made. Ultimately a common picture may emerge, seen in some instances of acute dilatation or toxic megacolon.

That the acute nature of the disease at the time of colectomy was responsible for the difficulties in histopathologic interpretation is suggested by the following figures. Twenty-seven of the 30 cases (90%) had required what can be described as urgent or emergency surgery.[17] The incidence of urgent or emergency surgery in the confidently indexed cases of ulcerative colitis was 40%, and in the cases of colonic Crohn's disease 2%, over the sample period. The figure is low for Crohn's disease in comparison with other papers as only surgical specimens were being considered, no biopsy data being included at this point.

In a retrospective survey it may be thought artificial to study the surgical specimen in isolation. In clinical practice, this is often the situation, especially in the urgent case and at a center dealing with referred material. By studying the problem from this aspect, along with the clinical correlations, an explanation for many of the diagnostic difficulties has emerged. Furthermore it becomes possible to fit these problem cases into the perspective of nonspecific inflammatory bowel disease. It has been shown that the histopathologist must be cautious in interpreting rectal sparing and an uneven disease pattern (Figs. 3 and 4) on the gross pathology without knowing the activity of the disease. Fissuring,

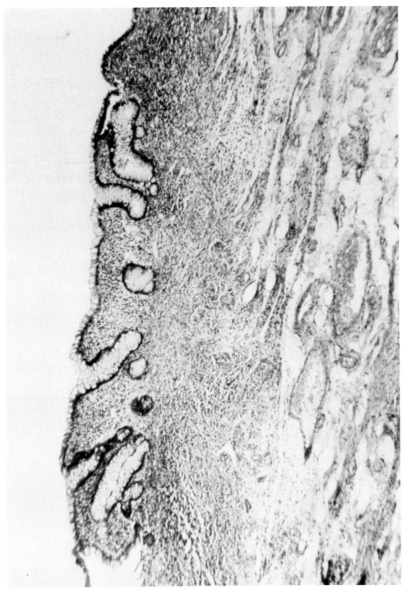

FIG. 10. Typical chronic ulcerative colitis in a quiescent phase. This is from a proctectomy specimen. Six months earlier an urgent total colectomy had been carried out and no definite diagnosis could be offered. Hematoxylin and eosin × 90.

transmural inflammation, the goblet cell population and the glandular pattern must also be carefully interpreted in the urgent operative specimen if mistaken classification is to be avoided.

Both Crohn's disease and ulcerative colitis are chronic diseases and while a demoralizing admission for a histopathologist, a definite diagnosis may not be possible at any given moment, even after examination of the operative specimen. Where possible a dynamic view of the disease process has to be taken and sequential biopsy, both preoperative and postcolectomy, must become part of routine management.

When the additional material available in these 30 cases was taken into account many of the difficulties were resolved. Biopsies were available prior to surgery in 23 of the 30 cases, and in 10 of these the rectum (6 cases), a rectal cuff (3 cases), or a rectal biopsy (2 cases) subsequently became available. A final confident diagnosis was made in 15 cases. Of these, 6 were classified as ulcerative colitis. This diagnosis was based on accepted histopathologic criteria,[11] absent or equivocal in the operative specimen because of the acute nature of the disease, yet seen in preoperative biopsies or postcolectomy tissue (Fig. 10). Nine cases with available preoperative or postcolectomy histology were finally classified as Crohn's disease. This was based on two main criteria, either the presence of granulomas, or the finding of normal rectal histology in postcolectomy cases that had long histories of nonspecific inflammatory bowel disease (Fig. 11). This was felt to be adequate grounds for a final diagnosis of Crohn's disease.

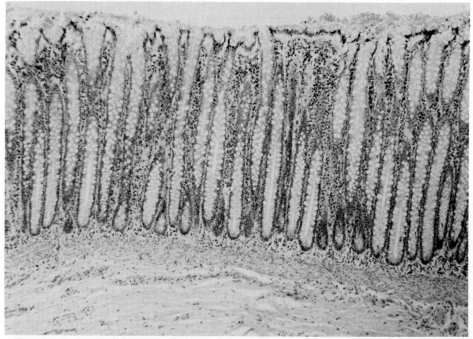

Fɪɢ. 11. Normal rectal mucosa. This is from a cuff of rectum excised at the fashioning of an ileorectal anastomosis. An emergency colectomy 1 year earlier was "unclassified." The normal histology is a strong pointer to Crohn's disease after this sequence of events. Hematoxylin and eosin × 90.

Significant histopathologic doubt remained in only 15 of the original 30 cases. In 7 of these no additional material was, or subsequently became, available for study.

CONCLUSIONS

The indeterminate nature of many cases of nonspecific inflammatory bowel disease, colitis unclassified, is the result of examining the surgical specimen at a moment in time when there is considerable overlap in the histopathology of Crohn's disease and ulcerative colitis, that is, during the development of their fulminant forms. The overlap is greatest in specimens removed at the time of established "toxic megacolon" or acute dilatation. The confusing features in diagnosis, which have been discussed, are because certain discriminating attributes, of importance in the less acute stages of the two conditions, become common to both in the developing fulminating state. These must be interpreted with caution if errors of classification are to be avoided. A qualified but clinically helpful diagnosis may have to be given in the acute severe phase.

Every opportunity for obtaining sequential biopsy material during less acute phases should be taken. When this is done many of the difficulties can be resolved and real diagnostic doubt will remain in only a small number of instances. A few unclassified cases will always remain, among the patients who require urgent or emergency surgery, until the etiologies of Crohn's disease and ulcerative colitis are discovered.

REFERENCES

1. Buzzard, A. J., Baker, W. N. W., Needham, P. R. G., and Warren, R. E.: Acute toxic dilatation of the colon in Crohn's colitis. *Gut 15:* 416–419, 1974.
2. Cook, M. G., and Dixon, M. F.: An analysis of the reliability of detection and diagnostic value of various pathological features in Crohn's disease and ulcerative colitis. *Gut 14:* 255–262, 1973.
3. Glass, R. E., and Baker, W. N. W.: Role of the granuloma in recurrent Crohn's disease. *Gut 17:* 75–77, 1976.
4. Glotzer, D. J., Gardner, R. C., Goldman, H., Hindricks, H. R., Rosen, H., and Zetzel, L.: Comparative features and course of ulcerative and granulomatous colitis. *New Engl. J. Med. 282:* 582–587, 1970.
5. Goodman, M. J., Skinner, J. M., and Truelove, S. C.: Abnormalities in the apparently normal bowel mucosa in Crohn's disease. *Lancet 1:* 275–278, 1976.
6. Hawk, W. A., and Turnbull, R. B.: Primary ulcerative disease of the colon. *Gastroenterology 51:* 802–805, 1966.
7. Jones, J. H. *et al.*: Numerical taxonomy and discriminant analysis applied to non-specific colitis. *Q. J. Med. 42:* 715–732, 1973.
8. Kent, T. H., Ammon, R. K., and Denbesten, L.: Differentiation of ulcerative colitis and regional enteritis of colon. *Arch. Pathol. 89:* 20–29, 1970.
9. Lennard-Jones, J. E.: Definition and Diagnosis: Regional Enteritis (Crohn's disease), pp. 105–112. In *Skandia International Symposia*, edited by Engel, A., and Larsson, T. Stockholm, Nordiska Bokandelns Forlag, 1971.
10. Lewin, K., and Swales, J. D.: Granulomatous colitis and atypical ulcerative colitis. Histological features, behavior and prognosis. *Gastroenterology 50:* 211–223, 1966.
11. Lockhart-Mummery, H. E., and Morson, B. C.: Crohn's disease (regional enteritis) of the large intestine and its distinction from ulcerative colitis. *Gut 1:* 87–105, 1960.
12. McGovern, V. J.: The differential diagnosis of colitis. In *Pathology Annual*, Vol. IV, edited by Sommers, S. C., pp. 127–158. New York, Appleton-Century-Crofts, 1969.
13. McGovern, V. J., and Goulston, S. J. M.: Crohn's disease of the colon. *Gut 9:* 164–176, 1968.

14. Morson, B. C.: Pathology of Ulcerative Colitis. In *Inflammatory Bowel Disease,* Ch. 12, edited by Kirsner, J. B., and Shorter, R. G., p. 176. Philadelphia, Lea & Febiger, 1975.
15. Morson, B. C., and Dawson, I. M. P.: *Gastrointestinal Pathology,* p. 269. London, Blackwell Scientific Publications, 1972.
16. Price, A. B., and Morson, B. C.: Inflammatory bowel disease. The surgical pathology of Crohn's disease and ulcerative colitis. *Hum. Pathol. 6:* 7–29, 1975.
17. Ritchie, J. K.: Results of surgery for inflammatory bowel disease. A further survey of one hospital region. *Br. Med. J. 1:* 264–268, 1974.
18. Roth, J. L. A., Valdes-Dapena, A., Stein, G. N., and Bockus, H. L.: Toxic megacolon in ulcerative colitis. *Gastroenterology 37:* 239–255, 1959.
19. Schachter, H., Goldstein, M. J., Rappaport, H., Fennessy, M. B., and Kirsner, J. B.: Ulcerative and "granulomatous" colitis—validity of differential diagnostic criteria. A study of 100 patients treated by colectomy. *Ann. Intern. Med. 72:* 841–851, 1970.
20. Sommers, S. C., and Korelitz, B. I.: Mucosal-cell counts in ulcerative and granulomatous colitis. *Am. J. Clin. Pathol. 63:* 359–365, 1975.
21. Whitehead, R.: Pathology of Crohn's Disease of the Colon. In *Inflammatory Bowel Disease,* Ch. 13, edited by Kirsner, J. B., and Shorter, R. G., pp. 286–287. Philadelphia, Lea & Febiger, 1975.

Chapter 2

Ischemic Bowel Disease: Its Spectrum

H. THOMAS NORRIS

Ischemic bowel disease refers to a spectrum of pathologic changes occurring throughout the gastrointestinal tract, caused by an abrupt decrease in blood flow through the intramural vessels of the bowel wall which produces focal ischemic changes initially in the mucosa. The ischemic process results in coagulative necrosis, with destruction of the mucosal barrier and subsequent invasion by bacteria. Although tissue anoxia is the common denominator, a single causative agent often cannot be implicated; rather, multiple contributing factors are usually necessary to cause pathologic change. In most cases, occlusion of the vessels supplying the ischemic area is absent or minimal. Depending upon the areas involved or the prominence of one of the etiologic factors, a variety of pathologic terms has been applied to the lesion. These include ischemic colitis, acute necrotizing enterocolitis of premature infants, hemorrhagic necrosis of the gastrointestinal tract, nonocclusive intestinal ischemia, hemorrhagic gastroenteropathy, pseudomembranous enterocolitis, Staphylococcal enterocolitis, radiation enterocolitis, ischemic enterocolitis, uremic colitis, potassium-induced stenotic ulcer, and stress ulceration of the gastrointestinal tract. This chapter will review the observations which resulted in the grouping of these disease processes under one heading. The causative factors, the pathophysiology, and the pathology of the lesions will be summarized.

It has only been during the last decade that reclassification of these lesions has occurred. An impetus to this reorganization has been the development of experimental models and new experimental techniques. It is not the intention of this chapter to exhaustively review the entire medical literature on the subject, but instead to cite those references which are particularly germane to the subject.

ISCHEMIC COLITIS

During the 1960's, Marston, Pheils, Thomas and Morson described three syndromes which result from ischemic processes of the colon.[16] These investigators pointed out that the clinical course is dependent upon three interdependent factors: 1) the degree of pathologic change in the visceral arteries supplying the colon, 2) the duration of hypotension, and 3) the virulence of bacteria present in the bowel lumen. In the most severe form, transmural gangrene of the colon results; in the intermediate form healing by fibrosis of the focally ischemic

15

colonic wall results in colonic stricture formation; the least severe form is characterized by episodes of bloody diarrhea with subsequent healing without sequellae. The pathophysiologic basis of these lesions is dependent upon enough blood being supplied to prevent complete death of the colon, with blood flow insufficient to meet the metabolic needs of the damaged mucosa. A combination of necrosis and subsequent bacterial invasion then occurs. While in the most severe form transmural gangrene develops, a more frequent presentation is infarction limited to the mucosa and submucosa.[7, 8, 9, 15, 36, 38] Ischemic colitis can occur anywhere in the large bowel.[13, 31] The region of the splenic flexure is most commonly affected. It is the anastomotic area between the colonic branches of the superior and inferior mesenteric arteries.

PATHOLOGY

The gross pathology of the most severe form is transmural infarction. Less severe forms show an ulcerated and hemorrhagic mucosa. If mucosal ulceration is extensive, pseudomembranes may be present (Fig. 1A). The serosal surface is actively inflamed in the gangrenous form; in less severe cases it is often uninvolved. Cross sections of the colon reveal an extensive hyperemia of the mucosa, and severe edema in the submucosa (Fig. 1B, C). The gross pathology of the intermediate form is a fusiform stricture, often 15 cm. in length. The mucosal surface has patchy superficial and longitudinal ulcerations. The submucosa is thickened due to fibrosis. Peritoneal adhesions are often present. The least severe form has a bluish-purple mucosal surface. Ulceration and active bleeding may be present.

MICROSCOPY

A sequential series of events is seen by light microscopy.[22, 23, 40] The earliest histologic changes occur in the most superficial mucosa.[5] Focal coagulative necrosis of the lamina propria is present with severe congestion of the microcirculation (Fig. 2A). These changes are immediately followed by extravasation of erythrocytes into the lamina propria. Occlusion of the blood vessels is not encountered. If the cause of the ischemia is not corrected, the process continues with involvement of the deeper portions of the mucosa, the submucosa and the muscular layer. Later stages reveal complete coagulative necrosis of the lamina propria with disruption of the surface epithelium and lamina propria. An acute inflammatory process is now present, with cryptitis and occasional crypt abscesses occurring in the mucosa (Fig. 2B). Pseudomembranes arise from the areas of mucosal damage, but may also cover less severely affected mucosa (Fig. 2C). The membrane is the result of extension of the acute inflammatory response into the lumen of the bowel, and is composed of necrotic mucosa, acute inflammatory cells, fibrin, and bacteria. The submucosa is edematous. The edema may be so severe that focal areas of mucosa and submucosa protrude into the lumen. These polypoid masses are transient in nature, and referred to as "thumb-prints" when seen on x-ray (Fig. 1B, C).

In cases presenting with stricture formation, marked fibrosis of the submucosal and muscular layers is present. The mucosa is ulcerated and replaced by granulation tissue. The principle feature of the least severe form of ischemic colitis is focal loss of the entire thickness of the mucosa with resulting ulceration. The submucosa is widened and filled with granulation tissue.

COMPARISON OF ISCHEMIC COLITIS WITH ULCERATIVE COLITIS AND CROHN'S DISEASE

While initially it was thought that ischemic colitis was a specific and distinct entity easily separated from ulcerative colitis and Crohn's disease, as more cases were studied this separation became less clear. Currently, no single finding is considered pathognomonic of ischemic colitis, ulcerative colitis, or Crohn's disease. The three conditions, however, can be distinguished on the basis of careful macroscopic and microscopic observations.[2, 24] As a general rule, ulcerative colitis spreads in continuity, beginning in the rectum, while Crohn's disease and ischemic colitis are regional or segmental in distribution. Ischemic colitis usually involves the splenic flexure. Pseudomembrane formation is common in the acute stages of ischemic colitis. It is absent in Crohn's disease and ulcerative colitis. A cobblestone appearance of the mucosa is seen in the acute phase of ischemic colitis and in Crohn's disease. Fissures which appear predominantly in Crohn's disease, and to a lesser extent in ulcerative colitis, are absent in ischemic colitis. The quality of the histopathologic response is quite different. Histopathologically, ischemic colitis is a process of coagulative mucosal necrosis and subsequent development of pseudomembranes. Crohn's disease is a transmural process with the consistent findings of edema, lymphocytes, and lymphoid nodules with germinal centers scattered throughout all layers. Ulcerative colitis is a mucosal histopathologic response with nonspecific crypt abscess formation, and in the acute phase, depletion of goblet cell mucus. Evidence of acute vasculitis or occlusion of the intramural vessels is usually absent in these cases. Vasculitis in the bowel wall is seen in patients with rheumatoid disease, systemic lupus erythematosus, dermatomyositis, and allergic phenomenon.

ACUTE NECROTIZING ENTEROCOLITIS OF PREMATURE INFANTS

During the mid-1960's, a reinterpretation of gastrointestinal complications of premature and low birthweight infants who had suffered severe perinatal stress occurred. Prior to this date, peritonitis, functional intra-abdominal abscess, spontaneous perforation of the ileum, appendicitis, and colitis with perforation were thought to be separate disease processes. It is now thought that these varied presentations are all manifestations of acute necrotizing enterocolitis.[11, 30, 32, 34, 35] The onset of acute necrotizing enterocolitis usually occurs in the 1st week of life. Three conditions must be present for susceptible infants to develop this disease: 1) the institution of feeding, 2) ischemic injury to the intestinal mucosa, and 3) the presence of bacteria in the lumen. Lesions have been reported in all segments of the gastrointestinal tract. The terminal ileum and right colon are most frequently involved. Occasionally, the entire colon and even the gastric wall may be involved. The pathologic findings are definitive. The time of examination and fixation of the specimen is imperative, however, as the earlier stages of this lesion mimic postmortem autolysis. At surgery, the involved segment is usually dilated and hemorrhagic, grey, necrotic and friable. Bubbles of gas (pneumatosis intestinalis) may be seen in the wall of the bowel

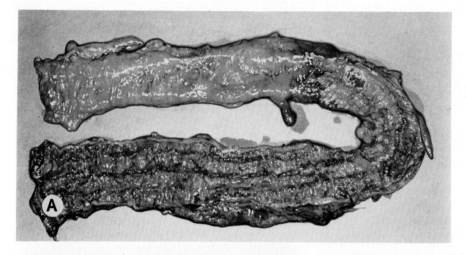

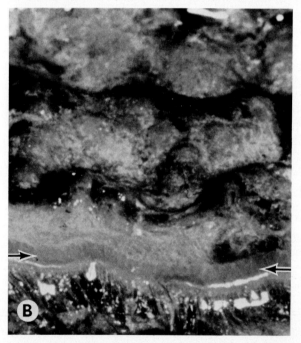

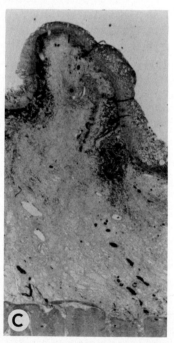

FIG. 1. *A*, gross photograph of mucosal surface of one type of ischemic bowel disease – ischemic colitis. The proximal one-third of the specimen is uninvolved. Just distal to the adenomatous polyp, the mucosa becomes ulcerated and is focally covered by pseudomembranes. *B*, close-up view of the layers of the bowel wall and adjacent mucosa. The entire mucosa is necrotic and focally covered by pseudomembranes. The distance between the muscular layer and the mucosa is greatly increased due to edema. The arrows indicate the position of the muscular layer. *C*, cross section of ischemic mucosa, submucosa and upper portion of the muscular layer of Figure 1*A*. The mucosa is completely infarcted. Between the mucosa and submucosa is a layer of congested vessels. Extravasation of erythrocytes in the submucosa is prominent. Edema may be focally very extensive, forming a polypoid projection into the lumen of the bowel. Hematoxylin and eosin, × 10.

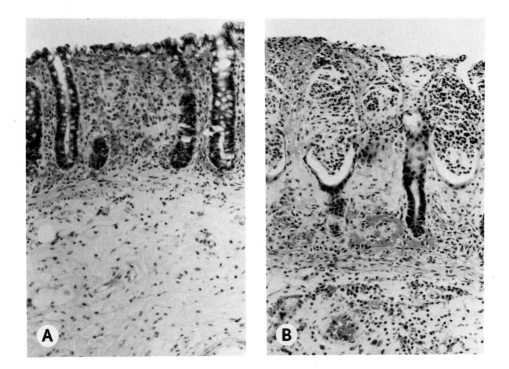

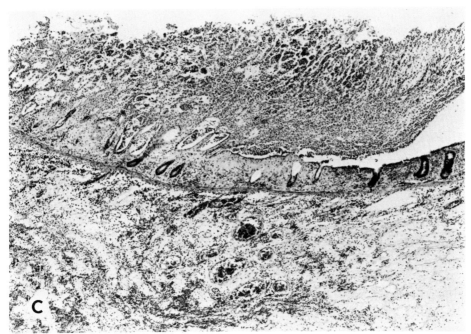

FIG. 2. A, early stage of ischemic colitis. Beneath an intact epithelium are severely congested vessels of the lamina propria. Slight extravasation of erythrocytes into the lamina propria is also present. The adjacent submucosa is edematous. Hematoxylin and eosin, × 140. B, later stage of ischemic colitis. The surface epithelium is denuded and the adjacent lamina propria is infarcted. The lower portion of the mucosa contains foci of acute inflammatory cells within the crypt lumina (cryptitis). The vessels of the adjacent edematous lamina propria are congested with focal extravasation of erythrocytes into the lamina propria. The underlying submucosa is edematous and contains acute inflammatory cells. Hematoxylin and eosin, × 140. C, Pathogenesis of pseudomembrane. Section of colon showing an infarcted mucosa on the left side of the figure, and a relatively intact mucosa on the right side. Pseudomembrane formation is a late finding, which results from the extension of the acute inflammatory process that has developed in the infarcted mucosa into the bowel lumen. The membrane is composed of acute inflammatory cells, fibrin and, occasionally, large numbers of bacteria. The submucosa is in the early stages of response to infarction, with severe congestion of the vessels and extravasation of erythrocytes into the edematous interstitium. Hematoxylin and eosin, × 88.

and the portal vein. Specimens that are not examined or fixed immediately lose some of their gross findings; in particular, the pneumatosis may no longer be seen (Fig. 3A). Infants who survive the acute episode may form benign strictures, which can occur as early as 5 weeks after the acute episode. The strictures usually occur either in the colon or ileum, and lead to subsequent intestinal

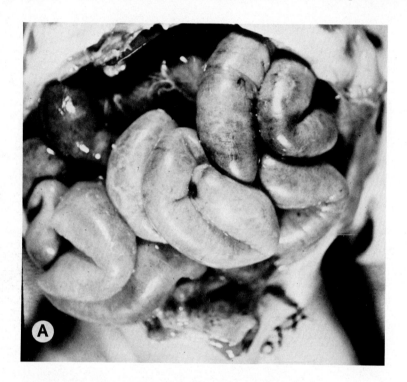

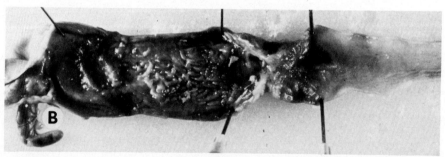

Fig. 3. *A*, gross photograph of autopsy findings in a patient with another type of ischemic bowel disease–necrotizing enterocolitis. The loops of bowel are dilated; well established infarction is seen in the loops in the right upper quadrant. Focally, the bowel is necrotic and friable. Pneumatosis, which was present earlier, has now disappeared. *B*, segment of right colon from a premature infant who died 12 weeks after an episode of necrotizing enterocolitis. Severe stricture formation is present in the ascending colon, with dilation of the proximal colon and ileum. Stricture is due to the deposition of fibrous connective tissue, especially in the submucosa and muscular layers.

obstruction (Fig. 3B). The initial recognition of the lesion occurred when fixation was obtained immediately following surgical resection (Fig. 4A). Microscopically, the earliest changes occur in the most superficial mucosa. Initially, coagulative necrosis is present with little inflammatory response. The vessels of the lamina propria are congested (Fig. 4B). As the lesion progresses, extravasation of erythrocytes occurs into the devitalized lamina propria (Fig. 4C). Superficial mucosal ulceration develops with eventual complete loss of the mucosa and severe ischemic changes extending into the submucosa (Fig. 4D). A grey pseudomembrane composed of necrotic epithelium, fibrin and inflammatory cells develops. Areas of impending perforation protected only by intact serosa are seen as well as areas of overt perforation. Little acute inflammatory response is seen until this stage has developed.

Now that the two ends of this spectrum have been examined, it is appropriate to consider some of the other presentations of this disease process.

HEMORRHAGIC NECROSIS OF THE GASTROINTESTINAL TRACT

Not all ischemic processes occurring in the gastrointestinal tract result in primary symptom complexes. In 1965, Ming[19] summarized cases of hemorrhagic necrosis of the gastrointestinal tract studied at autopsy, occurring as secondary phenomena in patients with severely compromised cardiovascular status, shock, or severe infection. Most of his cases were over 40 years of age. The associated clinical findings were shock, gastrointestinal hemorrhage, and abdominal complaints. Pathologic changes were similar in all cases, varying only in degree, severity, and extent of involvement. On gross examination, the mucosa was dark red with patchy or confluent areas of hemorrhage (Fig. 5A). Shallow ulcerations with necrotic bases were encountered. The serosa appeared purple or dark red, due to the large amount of blood in the lumen. The changes differed only from transmural infarction in that the serosa had a smooth surface and the adjacent mesenteric fat appeared normal. Thrombosis of major mesenteric vessels was noted only in 1 case. Microscopically, characteristic changes were seen and consisted of diffuse hemorrhage into the mucosa with coagulative necrosis beginning at the surface and extending downward to involve the entire mucosa (Fig. 5B). The necrotic process occasionally extended into the submucosa. The veins of the submucosa were markedly dilated. There were varying degrees of edema in the submucosa, however, only a mild neutrophilic reaction occurred in a few cases. While necrosis was common, gross membrane formation was rare. Evidence of mucosal regeneration was seen in many of the cases; this was characterized by pseudostratified glands with mitoses at the base of the crypts. Once again, the sparing of the muscular and serosal layers was present. Rarely, patchy necrosis of the muscularis propria was also encountered.[20]

OTHER PRESENTATIONS OF ISCHEMIC BOWEL DISEASE: PSEUDO-MEMBRANOUS, STAPHYLOCOCCAL, UREMIC AND RADIATION EN-TEROCOLITIS AND STRESS ULCERATION

It is unfortunate that some of these disease entities became inseparably associated with an etiologic factor, as all have pathologic changes similar to those just described.[2, 40] Pseudomembranous enterocolitis is so closely associated

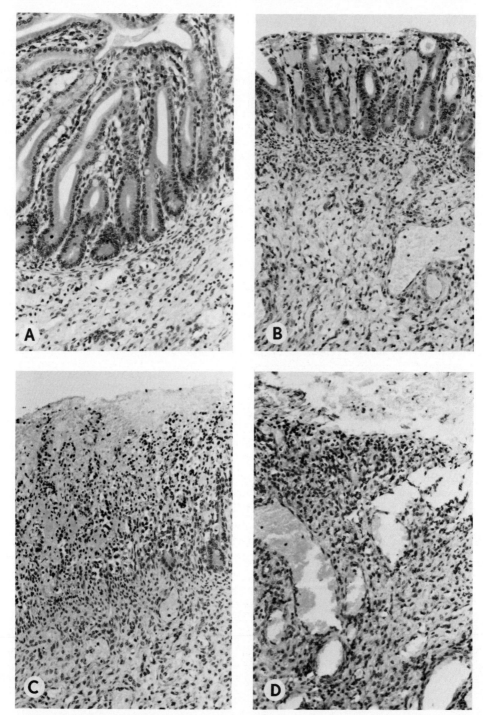

FIG. 4. Composite of the early stages of necrotizing enterocolitis occurring in the ileum. *A*, photomicrograph of the least-involved segment of the small bowel resected at surgery. Hematoxylin and eosin, × 140. *B*, earliest recognizable stage of necrotizing enterocolitis. The mucosa is atrophic with severe congestion of the superficial vessels of the lamina propria. The submucosa is also congested. Hematoxylin and eosin, × 140. *C*, later stage in the development of enterocolitis. The mucosa is infarcted with sloughing of the superficial portions. Remnants of crypts are present in the right side of the figure. The underlying submucosa is now severely congested. Hematoxylin and eosin, × 140. *D*, the mucosa is now completely sloughed. Congested and infarcted submucosa remains. The process will continue into the deeper layers of the bowel. An acute inflammatory response is not seen until the later stages of the disease process. Hematoxylin and eosin, × 140.

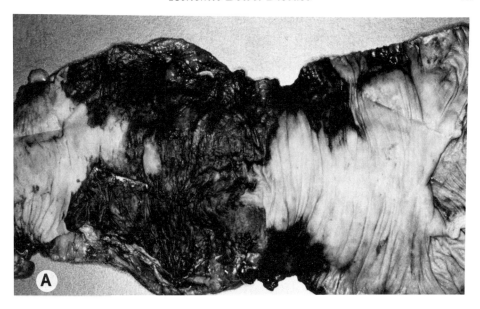

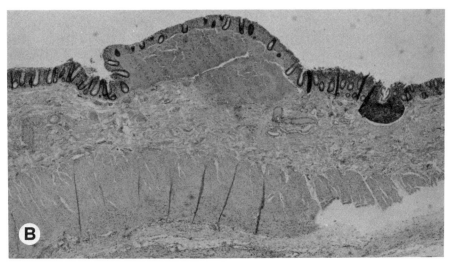

FIG. 5. *A*, gross photograph of the mucosal surface of another form of ischemic bowel disease—hemorrhagic necrosis of the intestine. Large areas of the mucosa are involved by hemorrhage and infarct. *B*, cross section of the early stage of hemorrhagic necrosis of the colon. Only a portion of the mucosa and submucosa is involved. The center one-third of the mucosal surface is infarcted with underlying congestion of the submucosa. Hematoxylin and eosin, × 20.

with antibiotic therapy or *Staphylococci* present in the bowel lumen that its possible ischemic basis has been overlooked, in spite of the fact that Penner and Bernheim,[26] in their original description, strongly alluded to this possibility. In Ming's series,[19] 20% of the patients had fatal infections, caused either by Gram-negative bacteria or coagulase-positive *Staphylococci*. Ming[19] and others[2, 10, 13, 26, 39] question the actual role of *Staphylococci* in the pathogenesis of this entity, and feel that pseudomembrane formation may be overemphasized. In addition, no experimental model using *Staphylococci* or its products will consistently cause the development of the pseudomembrane. No experimental model which uses ammoniacal toxic products for the production of uremic colitis has been successful. The morphology of these lesions is similar, if not identical, to that described in earlier paragraphs. The delayed changes seen in the colon following radiation, *i.e.*, fibrosis and partial obstruction of the bowel lumen, are also probably manifestations of an ischemic process. As proposed by Windsor,[41] when studying potassium-induced stenotic ulcers, patients with congestive heart failure may undergo periods of ischemia. The addition of potassium chloride may lead to more prolonged ischemia with hemorrhage, congestion, fibrosis, and eventual stricture formation in the small intestine. It is now apparent that the basic process underlying stress ulceration is hypoxic in nature.[17, 18, 33] Multiple shallow stress ulcers often develop in the upper gastrointestinal tract following a wide variety of stressful situations. Histopathologically, focal coagulation necrosis is the initial response to these lesions. (Fig. 6).

EXPERIMENTAL STUDIES

The described disease processes all share similar changes in the hemodynamics and consequently, the metabolic function of the gut. Techniques have been developed that measure the volume and the distribution of blood flow to the various layers of the gastrointestinal tract (Fig. 7). Over 50% of the microcirculation of the layers of the bowel wall perfused during normotensive conditions is not perfused during shock. Wolfe and Sumner[42] have recently measured the

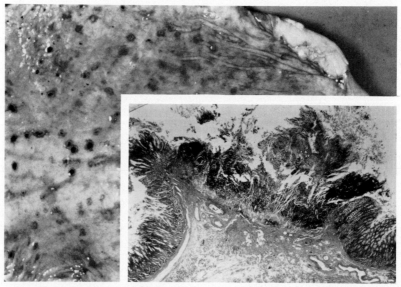

Fig. 6. Composite of stress ulceration of the stomach. Gross photograph demonstrates the various stages in the formation of stress ulcers, from focal mucosal congestion to complete loss of the mucosa. Insert is a section of gastric mucosa and submucosa showing focal coagulative necrosis of the mucosa and superficial submucosa. The underlying vessels are dilated. Insert hematoxylin and eosin, × 10.

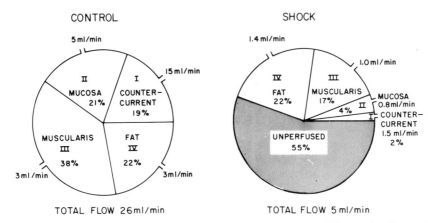

FIG. 7. Diagram of the distribution of blood flow to the layers of the canine ileum during normotensive conditions (control) and hypovolemic shock. The areas of the circle represent the amount of microcirculation which is perfused. Numbers at the periphery of the circle represent the volume of blood flow to each layer. During hypovolemic shock, over 50% of the microcirculation is not perfused. The volume of total blood flow is decreased by 81%. Only 19% of the microcirculation of the mucosa and submucosa is perfused during shock. The volume of blood flow to the mucosa and submucosa is decreased to 16% of control levels. In the muscular layer, the decrease in perfusion is 45% and decrease in the volume of blood flow is only 33% of control values. Courtesy of D. S. Sumner.

actual amount of capillary bed that is actively perfused, and the volume of blood flow through each layer of the small intestine during normotensive and hypotensive conditions. During shock, the amount of actively perfused microcirculation of the mucosa and submucosa is decreased to 19% of normotensive levels. The volume of blood flow during shock through the mucosa and submucosa is decreased to 16% of normal levels. During shock, the amount of actively perfused microcirculation of the muscular layer is decreased to 45% of the normotensive level, and the volume of blood flow is decreased to 33% of the normotensive level. These profound hemodynamic changes have been compared to the "diving reflex" of aquatic animals,[37] a reflex thought to protect the brain and heart from anoxia by shunting blood away from the mesenteric, renal, and peripheral vascular bed. In the lesions under discussion in this chapter, the period of hypoxia, however, is much more prolonged. Redistribution of blood flow is probably a specific response to hypoxia. Changes in blood flow distribution have not been studied in detail in other gastrointestinal conditions. When they were studied in an experimental model of human cholera, no changes in blood flow distribution were found, although marked physiologic changes had occurred in the mucosa.[25]

ISCHEMIC COLITIS

The most frequent site of involvement in ischemic colitis is the splenic flexure. Historically, this area of vulnerability was demonstrated after sacrifice of the inferior mesenteric artery during resection of aortic aneurysms. The splenic flexure reflects the watershed area between branches of the superior and inferior mesenteric arteries. The experimental counterpart of ischemic colitis utilizes complete occlusion of the vasculature for varying intervals.[4, 14, 28, 29] The results obtained closely resemble the clinical findings of the disease, and reiterate the relative susceptibility of the mucosa to anoxia when compared to other layers of the wall of the gastrointestinal tract. While different areas of the gastrointestinal tract show different susceptibilities to anoxia, once the lesion is established, these areas all respond in a similar manner. The ileum is more sensitive to anoxia than the colon, but also has a more rapid response to repair following restitution of circulation.

It is generally accepted that at least 1 hour of complete cessation of blood flow is needed to regularly produce the lesion in the colon. After this period of time, there is good agreement between the histopathology, the physiology, and the radiologic alterations obtained. After 1 hour of anoxia, net sodium transport across the colonic mucosa is abolished.[28, 29] Sodium and potassium ATPase levels are decreased after two hours of anoxia. At 1 hour, by light microscopy, remarkably little damage is observed. After three hours, the microcirculation has lost its integrity and there is extravasation of erythrocytes into the lamina propria. The degree of compromised microcirculation is even more evident if blood flow is reestablished before the colonic wall is resected for histologic examination. Marked submucosal edema and hemorrhage accompany the mucosal changes. Animals studied during recovery after three hours of ischemia revealed widespread destruction.[29] Following the initial stages of coagulative necrosis, the entire mucosa was replaced by hemorrhagic exudate containing polymorphonuclear leukocytes. The microcirculation of the muscular layer, however, remained intact and only minor and transient changes occurred in this layer.

The ultrastructural alterations are those typically encountered in acute ischemic injury, and can be observed as early as 15 minutes after the institution of anoxia.[1, 6] In addition, changes in the muscular layer are also observed on an ultrastructural basis.[20] The changes in the bowel wall can be delayed in experimental models ventilated with 100% oxygen.[1]

NEONATAL ENTEROCOLITIS

The experimental models used in neonatal enterocolitis are designed to simulate perinatal conditions.[3, 37] It is postulated that hypoxia may occur during delivery and the immediate postpartum period. The hypoxia causes decreased mucus formation and resultant mucosal damage. Bacterial invasion of the gut then ensues, unless passive enteric immunity (macrophages of breast milk) can control the gut flora. Production of the experimental lesion involves stressing the animal by a variety of methods, including asphyxia and exposure to cold.[3, 37] When the intramural and mucosal perfusion of the gut of asphyxiated and resuscitated neonatal piglets was compared,[37] no change in the total blood volume or total cardiac output was found. However, a marked reduction in blood flow both to the mucosa and the entire gastrointestinal tract occurred during asphyxia. Additional studies indicate that decreased perfusion is more severe in the stomach, distal ileum, and colon than in the duodenum and proximal and distal jejunum, suggesting the reason why perforation may be more frequent in the former sites than the latter ones. Multiple episodes of the stress were also important in the development of the lesion.[3] Other factors, including altered immunity and bacteria, have been implicated in neonatal enterocolitis.[3] Feeding experimental animals breast milk completely protected them from the development of the lesion following periods of stress, while those fed artificial formulas developed the lesion readily. The presence of pneumatosis is directly correlated with the presence of gas-forming organisms. While initial experiments utilized the addition of Gram-negative organisms, subsequent experiments revealed that the normal indigenous flora were sufficient to aid in the development of the necrotic bowel.

STRESS ULCERATION

The basic process underlying stress ulceration is nonocclusive focal ischemia. Using pO_2 tension as a measurement of the blood flow through the mucosa, Schellerer[33] demonstrated a marked decrease in the mucosal blood flow in animals stressed by a variety of methods. Menguy, Desbaillets, and Masters[17] have shown that severe gastric epithelial necrosis can occur within 15 minutes of nonlethal hemorrhagic shock, and that gross erosions occur within 45 minutes of this procedure. They speculate that an energy deficit hypothesis occurs. They have shown that the levels of available energy, fueled by adenosine triphosphate, are severely diminished in the affected gastric mucosa. This vulnerability may be related to the lack of oxygen in the tissues, and the relative inability of the tissues to utilize anaerobic glycolysis as an alternate source of energy. Menguy and Masters[18] have extended these findings and have shown that the nutritional state of the subject can also modify stress ulceration. More severe alterations occurred in the fasted animals as compared with the nonfasted animals. When fundus, corpus and antrum are compared, the energy deficit is more severe in the fundus and corpus than in the antrum.

In summary, during the last several years, advances in the understanding of the pathology and pathophysiology of ischemic bowel disease have occurred. Obviously, many questions remain unanswered. The role of many of the cellular components of the bowel wall is unclear; in particular, the role of the enterochromaffin cell and cells which play a significant role in other ischemic processes still needs to be ascertained.[14, 27] The role of other factors such as endotoxin and disseminated intravascular coagulation must also be pursued. Therapeutic approaches to modifying the extent of the lesion are also just being developed.

THERAPEUTIC IMPLICATIONS

Once ischemic bowel disease is diagnosed, therapy is devoted to correcting the abnormal pathophysiology. Recent studies indicate that experimental findings may be directly applicable to the clinical state. The fact that the lesions are a primary response to hypoxia is reinforced by the experimental finding that the functional and histopathologic consequences of this lesion can be postponed or inhibited by the administration of 100% oxygen.[1]

One of the dilemmas facing the surgeon during resection is the extent of involvement of the lesion. Previously used criteria such as return of color, bleeding, arterial pulsation and peristalsis are notoriously unreliable, requiring a "second look" procedure 24 hours following resection. This occurs especially in the very ill person or the patient with massive involvement of the gastrointestinal tract. The difficulty in localizing the injured segment is greater in the colon, where peristalsis can be very slow or erratic under laparotomy conditions. In addition, electromyography, surface temperature recordings, and frozen sections are notoriously time-consuming and unreliable. Recently, it has been shown that the viable gastrointestinal tract responds to revascularization procedures with reactive hyperemia of the intestinal vessels, *i.e.*, hyperemic perfusion of segments of injured bowel after circulation is restored. Reactive hyperemia can currently be measured by comparison of the rate of disappearance of intraarterially injected technetium-99m-labeled microspheres in injured and in normal gastrointestinal tract.[12, 21, 43] A ratio greater than 1 indicates hyperemia. The counting equipment has been modified so that procedures can be performed quickly and simply in the operating room.

The purpose of this chapter is to summarize the pathology and pathophysiology of a spectrum of diseases of the gastrointestinal tract, which all share tissue hypoxia as a common etiologic factor. For convenience, the entire group is referred to as ischemic bowel disease. Ischemic bowel disease occurs in all age groups from the premature infant to the elderly. The initial pathologic response is coagulative necrosis which begins in the mucosa, and if not resolved, continues through the entire width of the bowel wall. Later, an acute inflammatory response occurs and pseudomembranes may develop. Patients who overcome the acute phase often develop intestinal strictures. With increase appreciation of the disease entity, new therapeutic approaches have been developed which have significantly altered the natural history of the disease.

ACKNOWLEDGMENTS

E. A. Smuckler, M.D. provided helpful suggestions.

REFERENCES

1. Aho, A. J., Arstila, A. U., Ahonen, J., Inberg, M. V., and Scheinin, T. M.: Ultrastructural alterations in ischaemic lesion of small intestinal mucosa in experimental superior mesenteric artery occlusion; effect of oxygen breathing. *Scand. J. Gastroenterol. 8:* 439–447, 1973.
2. Allen, A. C.: A unified concept of the vascular pathogenesis of enterocolitis of varied etiology; a pathophysiologic analysis. *Am. J. Gastroenterol. 55:* 347–378, 1971.
3. Barlow, B., and Santulli, T. V.: Importance of multiple episodes of hypoxia or cold stress on the development of enterocolitis in an animal model. *Surgery 77:* 687–690, 1975.
4. Boley, S. J., Schwartz, S., Lash, J., and Sternhill, V.: Reversible vascular occlusion of the colon. *Surg. Gynecol. Obstet. 116:* 53–60, 1963.
5. Bounous, G.: Ischemic bowel disease; mucosal injury in low flow states. *Can. J. Surg. 17:* 434, 1974.
6. Brown, R. A., Chiu, C. J., Scott, H. J., and Gurd, F. N.: Ultrastructural changes in the canine ileal mucosal cell after mesenteric arterial occlusion; a sequential study. *Arch. Surg. 101:* 290–297, 1970.
7. Byrne, J. J., Wittenberg, J., Grimes, E. T., and Williams, L. F., Jr.: Ischemic disease of the bowel. II. Ischemic colitis. *Dis. Colon Rectum 13:* 283–289, 1970.
8. Clark, A. W., Lloyd-Mostyn, R. H., and Sadler, M. R. De C.: "Ischaemic" colitis in young adults. *Br. Med. J. 4:* 70–72, 1972.
9. Fagin, R. R., and Kirsner, J. B.: Ischemic diseases of the colon. *Adv. Intern. Med. 17:* 343–362, 1971.
10. Goulston, S. J. M., and McGovern, V. J.: Pseudo-membranous colitis. *Gut 6:* 207–212, 1965.
11. Hopkins, G. B., Gould, V. E. Stevenson, J. K., and Oliver, T. K., Jr.: Necrotizing enterocolitis in premature infants; a clinical and pathologic evaluation of autopsy material. *Am. J. Dis. Child 120:* 229–232, 1970.

12. Katz, S., Wahab, A., Murray, W., and Williams, L. F.: New parameters of viability in ischemic bowel disease. *Am. J. Surg. 127:* 136–141, 1974.

13. Kilpatrick, Z. M., Farman, J., Yesner, R., and Spiro, H. M.: Ischemic proctitis. *J.A.M.A. 205:* 74–80, 1968.

14. Manohar, M., and Tyagi, R. P. S.: Experimental intestinal ischemia shock in dogs. *Am. J. Physiol. 225:* 887–892, 1973.

15. Marcuson, R. W.: Ischemic colitis. *Clin Gastroenterol. 1:* 745–763, 1972.

16. Marston, A., Pheils, M. T., Thomas, M. L., and Morson, B. C.: Ischaemic colitis. *Gut 7:* 1–15, 1966.

17. Menguy, R., Desbaillets, L., and Masters, Y. F.: Mechanism of stress ulcer. IV. Influence of hypovolemic shock on energy metabolism in the gastric mucosa. *Gastroenterology 66:* 46–55, 1974.

18. Menguy, R., and Masters, Y. F.: Mechanism of stress ulcer. IV. Influence of fasting on the tolerance of gastric mucosal energy metabolism to ischemia and on the incidence of stress ulceration. *Gastroenterology 66:* 1177–1186, 1974.

19. Ming, S-C.: Hemorrhagic necrosis of the gastrointestinal tract and its relation to cardiovascular status. *Circulation 32:* 332–341, 1965.

20. Ming, S-C., and McNiff, J.: Acute ischemic changes in intestinal muscularis. *Am. J. Pathol. 82:* 315–326, 1976.

21. Moossa, A. R., Skinner, D. B., Stark, V., and Hoffer, P.: Assessment of bowel viability using 99^mTechnetium-tagged albumin microspheres. *J. Surg. Res. 16:* 466–472, 1974.

22. Morson, B. C.: Pathology of ischaemic colitis. *Clin. Gastroenterol. 1:* 765–766, 1972.

23. Morson, B. C.: Pathology of ischaemic colitis. *Bibl. Gastroenterol. 9:* 134–136, 1970.

24. Morson, B. C.: The pathology of colitis and other inflammatory diseases of the colon. *Deutsche Roentgengesellschaft, Refrante uber die Tagung 54:* 308–312, 1973.

25. Norris, H. T., and Sumner, D. S.: Distribution of blood flow to the layers of the small bowel in experimental cholera. *Gastroenterology 66:* 973–981, 1974.

26. Penner, A., and Bernheim, A. I.: Acute postoperative enterocolitis; a study on the pathologic nature of shock. *Arch. Pathol. 27:* 966–983, 1939.

27. Reichenbach, D. D., and Benditt, E. P.: Catecholamines and cardiomyopathy; the pathogenesis and potential importance of myofibrillar degeneration. *Hum. Pathol. 1:* 125–150, 1970.

28. Robinson, J. W. L., Rausis, C., Basset, P., and Mirkovitch, V.: Functional and morphological response of the dog colon to ischaemia. *Gut 13:* 775–783, 1972.

29. Robinson, J. W. L., Haroud, M., Winistörfer, B., and Mirkovitch, V.: Recovery of function and structure of dog ileum and colon following two hours acute ischaemia. *Eur. J. Clin. Invest. 4:* 443–452, 1974.

30. Rodin, A. E., Nichols, M. M., and Hsu, F. L.: Necrotizing enterocolitis occurring in full-term neonates at birth. *Arch. Pathol. 96:* 335–338, 1973.

31. Saegesser, F., and Sandblom, P.: Ischemic lesions of the distended colon; a complication of obstructive colorectal cancer. *Am. J. Surg. 129:* 309–315, 1975.

32. Santulli, T. V.: Acute necrotizing enterocolitis; recognition and management. *Hosp. Pract. 9:* 129–135, 1974.

33. Schellerer, W.: The role of mucosal blood flow in the pathogenesis of stress ulcers. *Acta. Hepatogastroenterol. (Sluttg) 21:* 138–141, 1974.

34. Stevenson, J. K., Oliver. T. K., Jr., Graham, C. B., Bell, R. S., and Gould, V. E.: Aggressive treatment of neonatal necrotizing entercolitis; 38 patients with 25 survivors. *J. Pediatr. Surg. 6:* 28–35, 1971.

35. Stevenson, J. K., and Stevenson, D. K.: Necrotizing enterocolitis in the neonate. In *Surgery Annual,* Vol. 9, edited by Nyhus, L. M. Appleton-Century-Crofts, 1976.

36. Sullivan, J. F.: Vascular disease of the intestines. Symposium on gastrointestinal physiology. *Med. Clin. North Am. 58:* 1473–1485, 1974.

37. Touloukian, R. J., Posch, J. N., and Spencer, R.: The pathogenesis of ischemic gastroenterocolitis of the neonate; selective gut mucosal ischemia in asphyxiated neonatal piglets. *J. Pediatr. Surg. 7:* 194–205, 1972.

38. Westcott, J. L.: Angiographic demonstration of arterial occlusion in ischemic colitis. *Gastroenterology 63:* 486–490, 1972.

39. Whitehead, R.: Reversible ischaemic colitis. *Practitioner 213:* 54–58, 1974.

40. Whitehead, R.: The pathology of intestinal ischaemia. *Clin Gastroenterol. 1:* 613–637, 1972.
41. Windsor, C. W. O.: Ischaemic strictures of the small bowel. *Clin. Gastroenterol. 1:* 707–717, 1972.
42. Wolf, E. A., Jr., and Sumner, D. S.: Redistribution of intestinal blood flow during hypotension. *Surg. Forum 24:* 20–22, 1973.
43. Zarins, C. K., Skinner, D. B., Rhodes, B. A., and James, A. E., Jr.: Prediction of the viability of revascularized intestine with radioactive microspheres. *Surg. Gynecol. Obstet. 138:* 576–580, 1974.

Chapter 3

Bacterial Enterocolitis

S. B. FORMAL AND P. GEMSKI, JR.

Two mechanisms have thus far been described by which enteric pathogens cause alterations in normal host function. In one process, as exemplified by *Vibrio cholerae* and some strains of *Escherichia coli*, the organisms must possess two attributes which are essential for them to produce disease. The bacteria must be able to multiply in the small intestine of the host, and, in addition, produce an enterotoxin which causes the epithelial cell to secrete water and electrolytes. Mucosal damage does not occur in these infections and as far as is known the colon is not involved in the disease process. On the other hand, other intestinal pathogens such as shigellae, salmonellae, and some *E. coli* strains must invade the bowel wall to produce disease. Mucosal damage occurs and the colon not only is affected but may be the primary site of infection. The mucosal alterations which are observed may range from an acute mild inflammatory response to gross ulceration, and it is the pathogenesis of these invasive infections which is the subject of this discussion.

The primary step in the invasive process is the penetration of the intestinal epithelial cell by the pathogen. Shigellae and salmonellae have been seen within the intestinal epithelial cells of experimentally infected animals using electronmicroscopic, fluorescent antibody and routine histologic techniques. Moreover with electron microscopy a general picture of the morphologic events of penetration has been developed. Because of sampling difficulties with shigellae, most sequential studies have been done with *Salmonella typhimurium*. The first observed host alteration following contact of the pathogen with the intestinal epithelium is a destruction of the brush border of the intestinal epithelial cell. The pathogen is then engulfed by means of an invagination of the cell membrane and is eventually contained in a vacuole within the epithelial cell. The integrity of the cell membrane and the brush border subsequently is repaired.[14]

Little is known of the properties which a bacterial cell must possess to penetrate the epithelium and no doubt several attributes are involved in conferring this ability. Since the initial event of penetration requires cell surface interactions between the organism and the host tissue, it seems reasonable to assume that the bacterial cell envelope is somehow involved in this process. Indeed there is some evidence to suggest that the chemical composition of the 0-

repeat-unit polymer of the cell wall lipopolysaccharide (LPS) somatic antigen can be one deciding factor in the penetration process. This conclusion is based on experiments in which *Shigella flexneri* hybrids, constructed by intergeneric mating, and expressing either *E. coli* 0-8 or 0-25 somatic antigens, were tested for invasive capabilities. Hybrids with the 0-8 antigen uniformly lost their ability to penetrate while some 0-25 hybrids retained their virulence.[3]

The avirulence of all the 0-8 *S. flexneri* hybrids may indicate that the chemical composition and structure of the 0-repeat unit is one determining factor for epithelial penetration by *S. flexneri*. Studies by Simmons[13] have revealed that the group antigenic determinants of *S. flexneri* 2a consist of a *N*-acetyl-glucosamine-rhamnose-rhamnose-rhamnose-repeat unit and that the attachment of secondary α-glucosyl side chains to this primary chain confers type 2 specificity. Similar studies on the chemical composition of *E. coli* 0-8 strains have shown that the immunodominant sugar of the 0-repeat unit is D-mannose. Thus, the 0–8 antigen determinant is chemically divergent from the *S. flexneri* somatic determinants. The possibility that chemical composition of 0-repeat units is a determining factor for epithelial cell penetration is given some support by the finding that *S. flexneri* expressing antigen 0-25 can conserve their penetrating ability and virulence. Although the chemical components of the 0-25 lipopolysaccharide layer have not been fully described, it has been established that rhamnose is present in its 0-repeat unit. Thus, although being serologically distinct, the 0-repeat units of the *S. flexneri* group antigens and the *E. coli* 0-25 antigen bear some chemical similarity. This may be reflected in the conservation of virulence by such 0-25 hybrids.

Factors other than the somatic antigen are also involved in penetration. This is best illustrated by colonial mutants of dysentery bacilli which lack the ability to invade. The wild type translucent (T) colony form penetrates while the opaque (O) form does not.[9] The relationship between this phenotypic change and the other changes in cellular properties of the O form remains unclear at the present time. The lack of significant differences in serologic properties and in gross LPS structure between the T and O derivatives excludes a smooth to rough mutation, which could account for the loss of virulence. In addition, neither the virulent T form nor its O derivative produce detectable pili *in vitro*. Nevertheless, significant increases in electronegative charge, in resistance to sodium lauryl sulfate, ethylenediaminetetraacetic acid (EDTA) and lysozyme, and the loss of sensitivity to some of the T coliphages all suggest some alterations in the cell envelope complex of the O form which have as yet to be defined. Because the initial event of penetration requires a cell surface interaction between the invading organism and the target epithelial cell, it is not unreasonable to consider that changes in the cell wall could be manifested as a loss in virulence.

Penetration of the epithelium by an organism is in itself not sufficient to cause overt disease. The pathogen must also be able to multiply in the host tissue. This conclusion is based on findings with a hybrid of *S. flexneri* which retained the ability to penetrate intestinal epithelium but lacked the capacity to multiply and persist in the mucosa.[1] Such strains produced a transient inflammatory reaction in the intestines of experimental animals which never progressed to signs of overt disease. Signs of disease were detected in volunteers but only after they were fed a dose exceeding 10^8 hybrid bacteria. These observations thus indicate that the severity of disease is determined at least in part by the extent of pathogen multiplication following the initial step of epithelial cell penetration. Efficient multiplication within these foci of penetration results in the evolution of the ulcerative lesions.

Following penetration and multiplication a complex of events occur which result in inflammation, ulceration, cramps, tenesmus, fever, and fluid loss. Investigations on some of these aspects of enteric diseases have been carried out for several years but studies on the mechanism of fluid loss caused by invasive organisms have only recently been initiated. It should be stressed that usually the fluid volumes are relatively small and rarely approach those of classical cholera. With the tissue damage that occurs in infections such as salmonellosis and shigellosis, one might expect that the diarrheal fluid is a transudate or exudate of the damaged epithelium. However, this does not seem to be the case, for in monkeys with active salmonellosis, permeability to small nonmetabolizable molecules such as erythritol and mannitol does not appear to be altered.[7] On the contrary other studies with *S. typhimurium*-infected rabbit ileum mounted in Ussing chambers have indicated that fluid is lost by an active secretory process.[2] This inference has been confirmed by perfusion studies in monkeys which were infected with either salmonellae or shigellae.[11, 12] In the case of those animals with shigellosis, secretion occurred in only the colon if the clinical disease was classical dysentery, *i.e.*, stools of small volume with blood, mucous, and inflammatory cells. However, in animals in which a watery diarrhea was a component of the syndrome, the jejunum, in addition to the colon, was observed to secrete. The secretion in the jejunum took place in the absence of any observable invasion by the pathogen or of histologic alterations.

Although this finding is suggestive of enterotoxin activity, enterotoxin production by highly virulent strains of either *S. flexneri* or *S. sonnei* has not been detected. On the other hand it has recently been shown that filtrates of *S. dysenteriae* do possess enterotoxic activity and it is likely that this is associated with the previously described neurotoxic and cytotoxic activities of this organism.[6] The role which this toxin has in the overall disease process is, nevertheless, not clear cut. Studies concerned with the disease-provoking capacity of a wild type *S. dysenteriae* 1 and genetic derivatives of it have been compared in several experimental models (rabbit ileal loop, starved guinea pig, monkey and man). These investigations reemphasize the importance of invasion in pathogenesis, since nonpenetrating mutants which were still toxin-producing failed to elicit overt signs of illness in either monkeys or man.[4, 10] These findings certainly do not exclude a function for Shiga toxin in the pathogenesis of Shiga dysentery. It is conceivable that enterotoxin elaborated after penetration by *S. dysenteriae* 1 could be a factor in pathogenesis and fluid loss. Some support for this is based on the observation that sera from patients with shigellosis can neutralize Shiga toxin, thus suggesting that toxin (in the case of *S. dysenteriae* 1) or antigenically related material (in the case of nontoxigenic shigella species) is produced *in vivo*.

On the other hand there is indirect evidence that an interaction of bacteria or bacterial product and the jejunum is a necessary prerequisite for the jejunal secretion which we have observed. This inference comes from experiments in which intestinal segments from clinically ill monkeys which had been challenged intracecally with *S. flexneri* were perfused.[8] A high proportion of animals challenged by this route exhibited signs of disease which might have started with mild diarrhea but which proceeded to classical severe dysentery. None of these animals exhibited the abnormalities in jejunal transport which were observed in diarrheal monkeys which had been challenged orally. These observations demonstrate that the classical dysentery need only affect the colon, but they also suggest that the watery diarrhea which may be a component of shigellosis may require the passage of bacteria through the small intestines. However, that mechanism which stimulates jejunal secretion is not yet known. Even though one cannot presently define a role for classical enterotoxin in invasive enteric pathogens in the area of the bowel where penetration does occur the end result may be similar to that of exposure of the intestinal surface to cholera or *E. coli* enterotoxin. In both instances an increase in concentration of mucosal adenyl cyclase is observed.[5] Thus in regions of penetration, fluid secretion may be mediated through adenylate cyclase in a manner similar to that which takes place in cholera infections.

This discussion has focused on the steps of penetration and fluid secretion in the overall pathogenesis of the invasive type of enteric infection. Certainly much more work in these areas is required and studies are progressing. Other signs of disease which result from penetration and multiplication in the bowel wall are fever, shock, cramps, and tenesmus. Research in the former two areas has been pursued for many years. However, little work has been addressed to the basic causes of cramps or tenesmus which may well result from an alteration in normal patterns of bowel motility. Techniques are now available to approach this problem, and, if only because of its potential practical importance, this area should be studied intensively.

REFERENCES

1. Formal, S. B., LaBrec, E. H., Kent, T. H., and Falkow, S.: Abortive intestinal infection with an *Escherichia coli-Shigella flexneri* hybrid strain. *J. Bacteriol. 89:* 1374–1382, 1965.
2. Fromm, D., Giannella, R. A., Formal, S. B., Quijano, R., and Collins, H.: Ion transport across isolated ileal mucosa invaded by salmonella. *Gastroenterology 66:* 215–225, 1974.
3. Gemski, P., Sheahan, D. G., Washington, O., and Formal, S. B.: Virulence of *Shigella flexneri* hybrids expressing *Escherichia coli* somatic antigens. *Infect. Immun. 6:* 104–111, 1972.
4. Gemski, P., Takeuchi, A., Washington, O., and Formal, S. B.: Shigellosis due to *S. dysenteriae* 1; relative importance of mucosal invasion versus toxin production in pathogenesis. *J. Infect. Dis. 126:* 523–530, 1972.
5. Giannella, R. A., Gots, R. E., Charney, A. N., Greenough, W. B., and Formal, S. B.: Pathogenesis of salmonella-mediated intestinal fluid secretion; activation of adenylate cyclase and inhibition by indomethacin. *Gastroenterology 69:* 1238–1245, 1975.
6. Keusch, G. T., Grady, G. F., Mata, L. J., and McIver, J.: The pathogenesis of shigella diarrhea. 1. Enterotoxin production by *Shigella dysenteriae* 1. *J. Clin. Invest. 51:* 1212–1218, 1972.
7. Kinsey, M. D., Formal, S. B., and Giannella, R. A.: Role of altered permeability in the pathogenesis of salmonella diarrhea (abstract). *Gastroenterology 68:* 926, 1975.
8. Kinsey, M. D.: Personal communication.
9. LaBrec, E. H., Schneider, H., Magnani, T. J., and Formal, S. B.: Epithelial cell penetration as an essential step in the pathogenesis of bacillary dysentery. *J. Bacteriol. 88:* 1503–1518, 1964.

10. Levine, M. M., DuPont, H. J., Formal, S. B., Hornick, R. B., Takeuchi, A., Gangarosa, E. J., Snyder, M. J., and Libonati, J. P.: Pathogenesis of *Shigella dysenteriae* 1 (Shiga) dysentery. *J. Infect. Dis. 127:* 261–270, 1973.

11. Rout, W. R., Formal, S. B., Dammin, G. J., and Giannella, R. A.: Pathophysiology of salmonella diarrhea in the rhesus monkey; intestinal transport, morphological, and bacteriological studies. *Gastroenterology 67:* 59–70, 1974.

12. Rout, W. R., Formal, S. B., Giannella, R. A., and Dammin, G. J.: Pathophysiology of shigella diarrhea in the rhesus monkey; intestinal transport, morphological, and bacteriological studies. *Gastroenterology 68:* 270–278, 1975.

13. Simmons, D. A. R.: Immunochemistry of *Shigella flexneri* O-antigens; a study of structural and genetic aspects of the biosynthesis of cell-surface antigens. *Bacteriol. Rev. 35:* 117–148, 1971.

14. Takeuchi, A.: Electron microscope studies of experimental salmonella infection. 1. Penetration into the intestinal epithelium by *Salmonella typhimurium*. *Am. J. Pathol. 50:* 109–136, 1967.

Chapter 4

The Pathology of Acute Nonbacterial Gastroenteritis*

JERRY S. TRIER, DAVID S. SCHREIBER, AND NEIL R. BLACKLOW

Acute infectious nonbacterial gastroenteritis is a major public health problem. Its frequency as a cause of illness in the United States is second only to the common cold.[6] In healthy, well nourished adults, the illness is generally self-limited, though often temporarily incapacitating, and results in significant economic loss as measured by lost work hours. More important, in infants and the aged and among malnourished populations in underdeveloped countries, acute infectious nonbacterial gastroenteritis is more serious and may be associated with substantial mortality as well as morbidity.

For many years, most studies of acute infectious nonbacterial gastroenteritis have been limited to the epidemiology and routes of transmission of the disease.[11, 12, 18] However, the recent identification and partial characterization of viral agents associated with acute infectious nonbacterial gastroenteritis have stimulated and made possible substantial additional research in this area. Two groups of viral enteric pathogens have been identified as probable major causes of infectious nonbacterial gastroenteritis: parvovirus-like agents which appear responsible primarily for disease in adults and older children[13] and reovirus-like agents which appear to be a major cause of viral diarrhea in infancy.[10]

As more became known about the agents causing nonbacterial gastroenteritis, the gastrointestinal pathology associated with these infections has been more clearly defined and some, albeit limited, progress has been made in defining factors which may or may not play a role in the pathogenesis of the clinical features.

ACUTE INFECTIOUS NONBACTERIAL GASTROENTERITIS IN ADULTS

There is evidence that several immunologically distinct parvovirus-like agents produce clinically indistinguishable disease in adults.[4, 8, 13] The two disease-causing agents which have been most extensively studied are Norwalk agent and Hawaii agent which were derived from outbreaks which took place in

* Supported by Grants AM-17537 and RR-00533 from the National Institutes of Health and by Contract DADA 17-72-C-2071 from the United States Army Medical Research and Development Command.

Norwalk, Ohio, in 1968 and in Honolulu, Hawaii, in 1971, respectively.[4] Both of these agents had been serially passaged through human volunteers. These agents appear as particles approximately 27 nm. in diameter in electron micrographs of stool filtrates which have been reacted with convalescent sera (Fig. 1). The clinical features of the illness produced in volunteers receiving bacteria-free filtrates containing Norwalk and Hawaii agents are summarized in Figure 2. Nausea, anorexia, malaise, headache, and myalgia are common. Vomiting and diarrhea may both occur in some infected volunteers with overt clinical disease, others may experience only vomiting without diarrhea while still others experience only diarrhea without vomiting. Transient low grade fever and leukocytosis may accompany the symptoms. The incubation period of the illness varies from approximately 12–48 hours and the duration of symptoms is usually less than 48 hours with vomiting, diarrhea, and other symptoms rarely lasting more than 12 to 18 hours.[4] In general, 40 to 80% of volunteers receiving an inoculum containing Norwalk agent or Hawaii agent develop clinically evident illness.

Peroral biospy studies of volunteers who have ingested an inoculum of Norwalk agent have shown that a characteristic mucosal lesion of the proximal small intestine regularly accompanies overt illness.[1, 21] In our studies, baseline biopsies were essentially normal (Figures 3A and 4A) in 12 volunteers who subsequently developed clinical illness upon ingesting Norwalk agent. In marked contrast, biopsies obtained 12 to 48 hours after ingestion of Norwalk agent during acute illness all showed a significant lesion which could be readily detected in coded slides which were randomized with the slides of normal pretreatment biopsies. The villi were shortened and the crypts were hyperplastic. The cellularity of the lamina propria was increased and it contained polymorphonuclear leukocytes as well as mononuclear cells. The villous absorptive

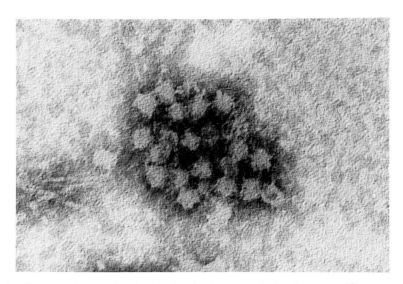

Fig. 1. Electron micrograph of stool filtrate from an adult volunteer with gastroenteritis caused by Norwalk agent. The filtrate was reacted with convalescent serum and negatively stained with phosphotungstic acid. The individual particles are irregular in outline and average 27 nm. in diameter. × 200,000.

cells were abnormal in all 12 patients (Figures 3*B* and 4*B*). Absorptive cell changes included patchy vacuolization of the cytoplasm (Figure 4*B*), decreased cell height, loss of nuclear polarity, and increased infiltration of the intercellular spaces between epithelial cells with mononuclear cells (Figure 4*C*).

Epithelial surface length of biopsies, a two-dimensional measurement which provides an indication of surface area, was quantitated in coded slides using a random point technique[19] and was substantively decreased from baseline levels in biopsies obtained from ill volunteers 2 days after administration of Norwalk agent (Fig. 5). In addition, the average number of mitotic figures in the crypt epithelium quantitated in coded slides was increased by more than 50% over baseline in ill volunteers 2 days following administration of Norwalk agent (Fig. 6). Biopsy abnormalities preceded the onset of clinical symptoms in some patients by as much as 36 hours.

Electron micrographs of biopsies obtained from patients ill with Norwalk agent disease have confirmed and extended somewhat the histologic observations.[1, 20] Abnormalities present in the absorptive epithelium include shortening of the microvilli, vacuolation of the cytoplasm, dilatation of the endoplasmic reticulum, swelling of the mitochondria, and accumulation of increased numbers of lysosome-like structures (Fig. 7). Clear-cut viral particles have not been identified in transmission electron micrographs of the intestinal mucosa.

Surprisingly, significant histologic abnormalities persisted in biopsies obtained 2 to 4 days after clinical symptoms had cleared (5 to 6 days after ingestion of Norwalk agent) in 10 of the 11 volunteers in our study. Architectural abnor-

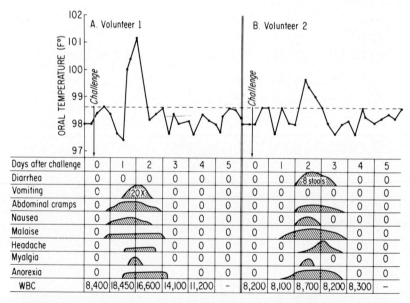

Days after challenge	0	1	2	3	4	5	0	1	2	3	4	5
Diarrhea	0	0	0	0	0	0	0	0	8 stools		0	0
Vomiting	0	20X	0	0	0	0	0	0	0	0	0	0
Abdominal cramps	0		0	0	0	0	0	0		0	0	0
Nausea	0		0	0	0	0	0	0		0	0	0
Malaise	0		0	0	0		0	0		0	0	0
Headache	0		0	0	0	0	0	0		0	0	0
Myalgia	0		0	0	0	0	0	0		0	0	0
Anorexia	0		0	0	0		0	0		0	0	0
WBC	8,400	18,450	16,600	14,100	11,200	–	8,200	8,100	8,700	8,200	8,300	–

FIG. 2. Response of 2 volunteers to oral administration of stool filtrate derived from a volunteer who received original Norwalk rectal swab specimen. The height of the shaded curve is roughly proportional to the severity of the sign or symptom. (Reproduced from R. Dolin, N. R. Blacklow, H. DuPont, S. Formal, R. F. Buscho, J. A. Kasel, R. P. Chames, R. Hornick, and R. M. Chanock: *Journal of J. Infectious Diseases 123:* 307, 1971.)

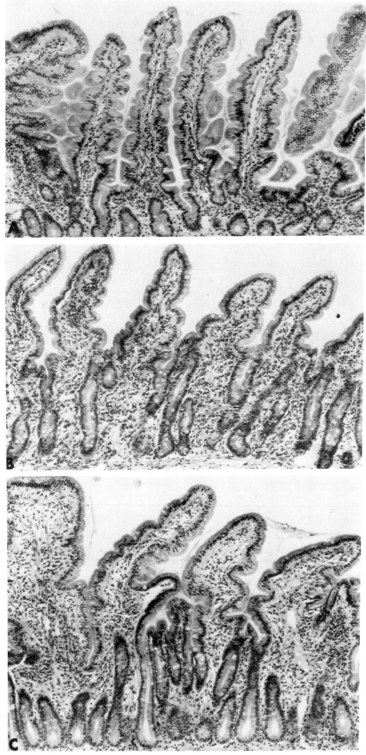

FIG. 3. Biopsies of the small intestine before and after oral ingestion of Norwalk agent. Before ingestion: *A* villi are tall, and the cellularity of the lamina propria is normal. Two days after ingestion: *B*, the villi are shortened, the crypts are hypertrophied and contain increased numbers of mitotic figures, and the cellularity of the lamina propria is increased. Six days after ingestion: *C*, shortened villi, hypertrophied crypts, and increased mitotic figures persist. Hematoxylin and eosin stain, × 100. (Reproduced from D. S. Schreiber, N. R. Blacklow, and J. S. Trier: *New England Journal of Medicine, 288:* 1318, 1973.)

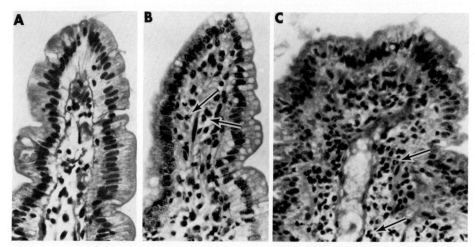

FIG. 4. Micrographs of villi. Before ingestion of Norwalk agent: *A*, tall columnar cells with compact cytoplasm and normal nuclear polarity are present. Cellularity of the lamina propria is normal. Two days after ingestion of Norwalk agent: *B*, the cytoplasm of epithelial cells from the same volunteer is vacuolated, and the cellularity of the lamina propria is increased and contains polymorphonuclear leukocytes (arrows). Another villus 2 days after ingestion: *C*, shows disordered nuclear polarity of the epithelial cells, increased numbers of mononuclear cells between epithelial cells, and extensive infiltration of the lamina propria, including polymorphonuclear leukocytes (arrows). Hematoxylin and eosin stain, × 350. (Reproduced from D. S. Schreiber, N. R. Blacklow, and J. S. Trier: *New England Journal of Medicine 288:* 1318, 1973.)

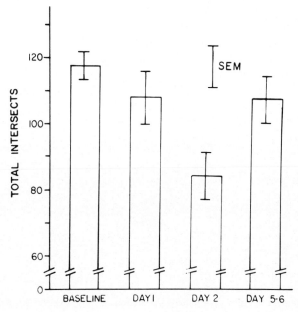

FIG. 5. Quantitation of the epithelial surface in intestinal mucosa before and after administration of Norwalk agent.

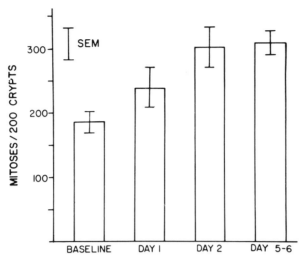

FIG. 6. Quantitation of mitoses in crypts in the small intestine before and after administration of Norwalk agent.

malities included villous shortening and crypt hypertrophy which was still striking (Fig. 3*C*) but mucosal inflammation and absorptive cell abnormalities were less consistent and, when present, less severe. The mean mitotic counts in crypts were still strikingly elevated (Fig. 6) but mean surface length had reverted toward normal (Fig. 5). Biopsies obtained 6 or more weeks after symptoms had cleared were entirely normal.

In some volunteers who remained asymptomatic after ingesting Norwalk agent sequential intestinal biopsies remained entirely normal. In others, significant lesions indistinguishable from those seen in symptomatic subjects developed 1 to 2 days after ingestion of the inoculum,[21] indicating that infection with intestinal histologic lesions can develop in the absence of clinically overt illness.

Inocula containing Hawaii agent induce a mucosal lesion in the proximal small intestine of volunteers who become symptomatic which is histologically indistinguishable from the lesion induced by Norwalk agent.[8, 22] As with Norwalk agent, some volunteers who remain asymptomatic after receiving Hawaii agent develop a typical intestinal mucosal lesion; others show no histologic alteration in sequentially obtained intestinal biopsies.[22] As in Norwalk agent-induced disease, nonspecific ultrastructural changes are seen in intestinal cells during illness induced by Hawaii agent, but viral particles have not been identified within mucosal cells.[8]

Although the histologic features of the lesion of the proximal mucosa of the small intestine induced by Norwalk and Hawaii agents are characteristic, the lesion is not specific. For example, histologic changes which appear virtually identical can be seen in patients with tropical sprue and intraluminal bacterial overgrowth (Fig. 8).

Volunteers who develop clinical illness following ingestion of Norwalk agent do not develop a histologically detectable gastric mucosal lesion.[24] Serial biop-

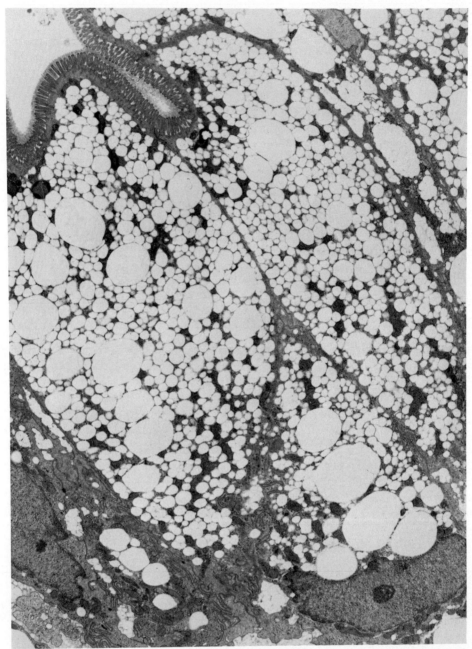

Fig. 7. Electron micrograph of intestinal epithelial cells from a biopsy obtained 36 hours after administration of Norwalk agent. There is extensive cytoplasmic vacuolization and the microvilli are decreased in height. × 4200.

sies of gastric fundus and/or gastric antrum in 9 volunteers who developed symptoms after ingesting Norwalk agent showed no significant histologic changes from baseline biopsies during acute illness and the immediate period of convalescence (Fig. 9 and 10). Gastric mucosal architecture, degree of inflammation in the lamina propria, and the cytology of epithelial cell elements remained unchanged during acute illness.

The pathophysiology of the symptoms associated with Norwalk agent- and Hawaii agent-induced disease remains to be clarified. Transient steatorrhea,[4] xylose malabsorption,[4, 21] and brush border disaccharidase deficiency[1] have been documented during acute illness induced by Norwalk agent. On the other hand, adenylate cyclase levels in the proximal intestinal mucosa do not increase during acute illness induced by either Norwalk agent or Hawaii agent.[16] Studies of fluid and electrolyte transport in disease caused by these agents have not been reported. Moreover, it has not been established whether the lesion which consistently involves the proximal small intestine is also present in the more distal small intestine.

The fact that vomiting frequently accompanies Norwalk agent-induced disease in the absence of a histologically detectable gastric mucosal lesion[24] is of interest. However, it has recently been shown that experimentally induced intestinal mucosal lesions in rats result in marked gastric retention.[15] Since we have observed that a number of patients vomit the remains of a meal eaten as long as 16 hours earlier during both Norwalk agent- and Hawaii agent-induced illness, it may be that impaired gastric motor function may play a major role in the pathogenesis of the vomiting frequently seen in acute infectious nonbacterial gastroenteritis.

ACUTE INFECTIOUS NONBACTERIAL GASTROENTERITIS IN INFANTS

There is increasing evidence that a human reovirus-like agent (HRVL) quite different from the parvovirus-like agent found in adults is responsible for a

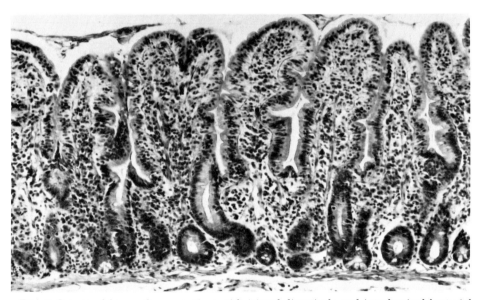

FIG. 8. Intestinal biopsy from a patient with jejunal diverticula and intraluminal bacterial overgrowth. The histologic alterations resemble closely those observed during gastroenteritis induced by Norwalk and Hawaii agents. × 140.

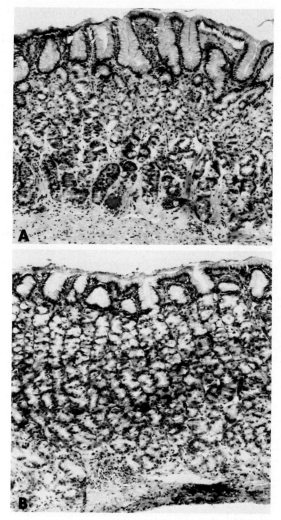

Fig. 9. Light micrographs of gastric fundal mucosal biopsies from a volunteer before (*A*) and during clinical illness (*B*) induced by Norwalk agent. Both biopsies appear normal. Hematoxylin and eosin stain, × 100. (Reproduced from L. Widerlite, J. S. Trier, N. R. Blacklow, and D. S. Schreiber: *Gastroenterology 68:* 425, 1975.)

substantial percentage of cases of acute gastroenteritis in infants and young children. Information regarding HRVL-induced gastroenteritis has been derived largely from studies of naturally occurring disease in infants and young children, unlike adult disease produced by parvovirus-like agents which has been studied experimentally under controlled conditions. Since its morphologic features[17] and immunologic characteristics[10, 14] differ from known reoviruses, the causative HRVL has been termed an orbivirus,[3, 17] rotavirus,[9] and duovirus[5] by different investigators. The HRVL particles are substantially larger than the parvovirus-like particles and have a diameter of approximately 60–70 nm. but larger-sized enveloped particles have also been described in tissue[3] (Figs. 11 and

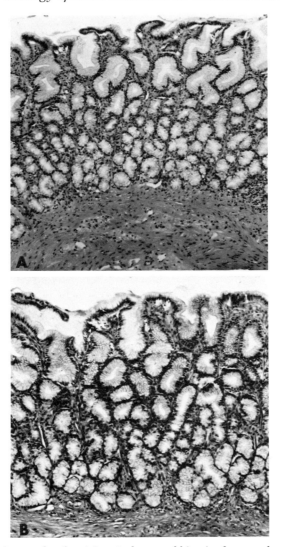

FIG. 10. Light micrographs of gastric antral mucosal biopsies from a volunteer before (*A*) and during clinical illness (*B*) induced by Norwalk agent. Both biopsies appear normal. Hematoxylin and eosin stain, × 100. (Reproduced from L. Widerlite, J. S. Trier, N. R. Blacklow, and D. S. Schreiber: *Gastroenterology 68:* 425, 1975.)

12). Infection with this agent is much more common during the winter and spring months than during summer and fall, and appears responsible for approximately 50% of acute gastroenteritis observed during the first 2 to 3 years of life. Clinically overt gastroenteritis due to HRVL in adults appears to be uncommon although apparent disease was produced in a single adult volunteer by intraduodenal challenge with this agent.[17] The incidence of asymptomatic infection with HRVL in children and in adults is not known.

Infection can be documented by visualizing the HRVL particles by electron microscopy by negative staining of stool suspensions with or without prior

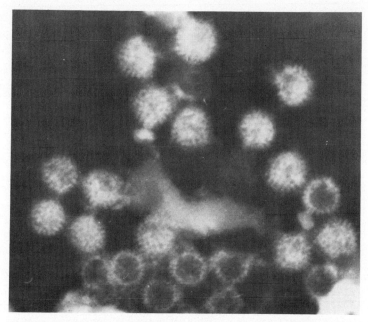

Fig. 11. Electron micrograph of stool suspension from an infant with gastroenteritis. Human reovirus-like particles are evident in this negatively stained preparation. The particles average approximately 65 nm. in diameter. × 160,000.

exposure of the stool to convalescent sera (Fig. 11). In contrast to infection induced by parvovirus-like agents, a reliable complement fixation test has been developed for HRVL in which stool filtrates of infected patients or the Nebraska calf diarrhea virus serve as antigens.[14] A rise in antibody titer in sera obtained during convalescence compared to sera obtained during acute illness indicates infection with HRVL. Moreover, while convincing evidence of *in vitro* cultivation of parvovirus-like agents is not available, HRVL associated with nonbacterial infantile gastroenteritis has recently been propagated in human fetal intestinal organ culture.[25]

Though available studies are limited, the histologic lesion seen in the proximal small intestine of infants and children with naturally occurring HRVL infections appears similar to the lesion seen in adults. Shortening of villi, infiltration of the lamina propria with increased numbers of plasma cells, and patchy abnormalities of villous epithelial cells have been described.[2] Intestinal mucosal disaccharidase levels are also decreased in biopsies during gastroenteritis associated with HRVL. Whereas viral particles have not been identified in the abnormal intestinal mucosa in Norwalk agent- or Hawaii agent-induced gastroenteritis, HRVL particles have been demonstrated in tissue sections of intestinal epithelial cells[3, 23] (Fig. 12) and in cells in the lamina propria[23] of ill infants by electron microscopy. Moreover, viral antigen has been demonstrated in HRVL gastroenteritis by indirect immunofluorescence in epithelial cells of the small intestine with sera from infected patients and antiserum raised in a guinea pig using particle-containing stool concentrate.[5, 17]

There is no published data to indicate that a gastric mucosal lesion accompan-

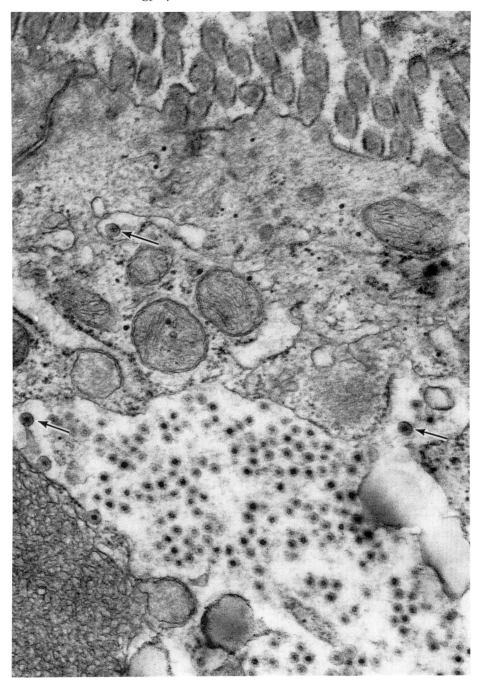

Fɪɢ. 12. Thin section electron micrograph of an intestinal epithelial cell in a biopsy specimen from a child with acute gastroenteritis. Numerous virus particles are seen in dilated cisterns of endoplasmic reticulum. Arrows indicate larger, enveloped particles. (Reproduced from R. F. Bishop, G. P. Davidson, I. H. Holmes, and B. J. Ruck: *Lancet 2:* 1281, 1973.)

ies the small intestinal lesion in HRVL-induced gastroenteritis. Whether or not the large intestine is involved is not known.

CONCLUSION

It is clear that the causative viruses of most cases of acute infectious nonbacterial gastroenteritis differ in adults and older children compared to infants and young children. In adults and older children, parvovirus-like agents have been found causative whereas in infants and young children a human reovirus-like agent has been implicated. Both produce a significant, though nonspecific, histologic lesion characterized by shortened villi, hyperplastic crypts, abnormal villous absorptive cells, and inflammation of the lamina propria. Virus-like particles have been identified by electron microscopy in the mucosa of infants and young children with disease due to human reovirus-like agents but not in the mucosa of adults infected with parvovirus-like agents. Asymptomatic infection with a characteristic proximal intestinal lesion has been documented in adults. There is no histologic lesion of the stomach in infected adults whereas the available data regarding gastric mucosal histology in infected infants and young children is too limited to be conclusive. Similarly, available data regarding possible colonic involvement in acute infectious nonbacterial gastroenteritis is limited and inconclusive. Finally, the extent of involvement of the small intestine by the characteristic lesion is unknown since only mucosa of the proximal small intestine has been studied.

REFERENCES

1. Agus, S. G., Dolin, R., Wyatt, R. G., Tousimis, A. J., and Northrup, R. S.: Acute infectious nonbacterial gastroenteritis; intestinal histopathology. *Ann. Intern. Med. 79:* 18–25, 1973.
2. Barnes, G. L., and Townley, R. R. W: Duodenal mucosal damage in 31 infants with gastroenteritis. *Arch. Dis. Child. 48:* 343–349, 1973.
3. Bishop, R. F., Davidson, G. P., Holmes, I. H., and Ruck, B. J.: Virus particles in epithelial cells of duodenal mucosa from children with acute non-bacterial gastroenteritis. *Lancet 2:* 1281–1283, 1973.
4. Blacklow, N. R., Dolin, R., Fedson, D. S., DuPont, H., Northrup, R. S., Hornick, R. B., and Chanock, R. M.: Acute infectious nonbacterial gastroenteritis; etiology and pathogenesis. *Ann. Intern. Med. 76:* 993–1008, 1972.
5. Davidson, G. P., Goller, I., Bishop, R. F., Townley, R. R. W., Holmes, I. H., and Ruck, B. J.: Immunofluorescence in duodenal mucosa of children with acute enteritis due to a new virus. *J. Clin Pathol. 28:* 263–266, 1975.
6. Dingle, J. H., Badger, G. F., Feller, A. E., Hodges, R. G., Jordan, W. S., and Rammelkamp, C. H.: A study of illness in a group of Cleveland families. I. Plan of study and certain general observations. *Am. J. Hyg. 58:* 16–30, 1953.
7. Dolin, R., Blacklow, N. R., DuPont, H., Formal, S., Buscho, R. F., Kasel, J. A., Chames, R. P., Hornick, R., and Chanock, R. M.: Transmission of acute infectious nonbacterial gastroenteritis to volunteers by oral administration of stool filtrates. *J. Infect. Dis. 123:* 307–312, 1971.
8. Dolin, R., Levy, A. G., Wyatt, R. G., Thornhill, T. S., and Gardner, J. D.: Viral gastroenteritis induced by the Hawaii agent. Jejunal histopathology and serologic response. *Am. J. Med. 59:* 761–768, 1975.
9. Flewett, T. H., Bryden, A. S., Davies, H., Woode, G. N., Bridger, J. C., and Derrick, J. M.: Relation between viruses from acute gastroenteritis of children and newborn calves. *Lancet 2:* 61–63, 1974.
10. Flewett, T. H., Bryden, A. S., and Davies, H.: Diagnostic electron microscopy faeces. I. The viral flora of the faeces as seen by electron microscopy. *J. Clin. Pathol. 27:* 603–614, 1974.

11. Gordon, I., Ingraham, H. S., and Korns, R. F.: Transmission of epidemic gastroenteritis to human volunteers by oral administration of fecal filtrates. *J. Exp. Med. 86:* 409–422, 1947.

12. Jordan, W. S., Gordon, I., and Dorrance, W. R.: A study of illness in a group of Cleveland families. VII. Transmission of acute non-bacterial gastroenteritis to volunteers; evidence for two different etiologic agents. *J. Exp. Med. 98:* 461–475, 1953.

13. Kapikian, A. Z., Wyatt, R. G., Dolin, R., Thornhill, T. S., Kalica, A. R., and Chanock, R. M.: Visualization by immune electron microscopy of a 27-nm particle associated with acute infectious nonbacterial gastroenteritis. *J. Virol. 10:* 1075–1081, 1972.

14. Kapikian, A. Z., Kim, H. W., Wyatt, R. G., Rodriguez, W. J., Ross, S., Cline, W. L., Parrott, R. H., and Chanock, R. M.: Reovirus-like agent in stools; association with infantile diarrhea and development of serologic tests. *Science 185:* 1049–1053, 1974.

15. Kent, T. H., Cannon, B., Reynolds, J., and Osborne, J. W.: Gastric emptying and small intestinal mucosal injury in rats. *Gastroenterology 69:* 1246–1253, 1975.

16. Levy, A. G., Widerlite, L., Schwartz, C. J., Dolin, R., Blacklow, N. R., Gardner, J. D., Kimberg, D. V., and Trier, J. S.: Jejunal adenylate cyclase activity in human subjects during viral gastroenteritis. *Gastroenterology 70:* 321–325, 1976.

17. Middleton, P. J., Szymanski, M. T., Abbott, G. D., Bortolussi, R., and Hamilton, J. R.: Obivirus gastroenteritis of infancy. *Lancet 1:* 1241–1244, June 22, 1974.

18. Reimann, H. A., Price, A. H., and Hodges, J. H.: The cause of epidemic diarrhea, nausea and vomiting (viral dysentery?). *Proc. Soc. Exp. Biol. Med. 59:* 8–9, 1945.

19. Rubin, C. E., Brandborg, L. L., Phelps, P. C., and Taylor, H. C.: Studies of celiac disease. I. The apparent identical and specific nature of the duodenal and proximal jejunal lesion in celiac disease and idiopathic sprue. *Gastroenterology 38:* 28–49, 1960.

20. Schreiber, D., Blacklow, N., and Trier, J.: The intestinal lesion in acute nonbacterial gastroenteritis (ANG) (abstract). *Clin. Res. 21:* 524, 1973.

21. Schreiber, D. S., Blacklow, N. R., and Trier, J. S.: The mucosal lesion of the proximal small intestine in acute infectious nonbacterial gastroenteritis. *N. Engl. J. Med. 288:* 1318–1323, 1973.

22. Schreiber, D. S., Blacklow, N. R., and Trier, J. S.: The small intestinal lesion induced by Hawaii agent acute infectious nonbacterial gastroenteritis. *J. Infect. Dis. 129:* 705–708, 1974.

23. Suzuki, H., and Konno, T.: Reovirus-like particles in jejunal mucosa of a Japanese infant with acute infectious non-bacterial gastroenteritis. *Tohoku J. Exp. Med. 115:* 199–211, 1975.

24. Widerlite, L., Trier, J. S., Blacklow, N. R., and Schreiber, D. S.: Structure of the gastric mucosa in acute infectious nonbacterial gastroenteritis. *Gastroenterology 68:* 425–430, 1975.

25. Wyatt, R. G., Kapikian, A. Z., Thornhill, T. S., Sereno, M. M., Kim, H. W., and Chanock, R. M.: In vitro cultivation in human fetal intestinal organ culture of a reovirus-like agent associated with nonbacterial gastroenteritis in infants and children. *J. Infect. Dis. 130:* 523–528, 1974.

Chapter 5

Colo-Rectal Biopsy in Inflammatory Bowel Disease

JOHN H. YARDLEY AND MARK DONOWITZ

The term inflammatory bowel disease (IBD) encompasses a large group of inflammatory disorders of the small and large intestine, most of which result from known infectious agents, toxic substances, and intrinsic abnormalities (see Table 2, below). The term is also used in a narrower sense to refer only to ulcerative colitis and to Crohn's disease,[41, 75, 80] but we prefer to designate those two entities by a modified term such as chronic idiopathic IBD or simply idiopathic IBD. This is not just a matter of accuracy for its own sake. The habit of using a more explicit term to cover collectively ulcerative colitis and Crohn's disease serves as a reminder that IBD has a broad, incompletely explored range of diagnostic possibilities, and also tends to increase the likelihood that treatable forms of IBD will be sought out when dealing with individual patients.

Since the large intestine is frequently involved in IBD, and since it is also accessible for biopsy, the colon, and especially the rectum, are the chief sources of tissue for diagnosis and follow-up study. Increasing numbers of colo-rectal biopsies are being obtained for these purposes, particularly since the advent of colonoscopy. On the other hand, it is our experience that pathologists often fail to make optimal interpretations of colo-rectal biopsies from patients with IBD. Optimal interpretation depends on the use of adequate methods for preparing the biopsy samples, familiarity with the basic histologic findings in normal and abnormal material, and the use of a systematic approach to the differential diagnostic possibilities. All of these aspects will be considered in this chapter.

A variety of monographs, articles, and brief summaries dealing with IBD and with interpretation of colo-rectal biopsies in IBD are available and should be helpful to the reader.[16, 20, 34, 41, 55, 56, 57]

TECHNICAL CONSIDERATIONS

The choice of fixatives often depends on local conditions and personal preference, and many pathologists feel that 10% formalin in saline, buffered to pH 7, gives perfectly satisfactory fixation of colo-rectal biopsies. In our experience, however, ordinary formalin causes excessive loss of detail because of shrinkage. Fixatives of the Helly's type give better results, but are complicated to use, since mixing just prior to use and careful timing of the fixation period are necessary. Bouin's fixative and formol-mercury are preferred in some laboratories and give good results.

The fixative which we employ for colo-rectal biopsies (as well as all other biopsies of the gastrointestinal tract) gives results similar to those obtained with the Bouin's solution. The fixative, which was originated by Moore, Graham, and Barr[53] has the following formulation: acetic acid (glacial), 100 ml.; formalin (100%), 200 ml.; alcohol (95%), 350 ml.; and water, 350 ml.; total, 1000 ml.

This fixative has an indefinite shelf life and requires no special procedures for its use. Nuclear and cytoplasmic detail are well preserved, and there is minimal shrinkage of the type usually encountered with plain formalin. The most significant disadvantage of the acetic acid-formalin-alcohol mixture is that granules of eosinophils and Paneth cells are lysed so that additional biopsies must be placed in neutral buffered formalin or other appropriate fixative if these features are to be studied.

The accuracy and completeness with which colo-rectal biopsies can be interpreted are greatly increased by orienting the specimens so that they are sectioned perpendicular to the mucosa. Orientation is assisted by spreading the specimen, mucosa up, on a substrate of nylon mesh, Gelfoam, a piece of frosted glass, slice of cucumber, or other suitable material prior to fixation. This approach works well when it is properly done, but it is less practical with the smaller specimens obtained through the colonoscope. Problems are also encountered when several persons in a busy endoscopy service, some of whom are almost inevitably inexperienced, are responsible for orienting the specimens. The mucosa is easily damaged by rough handling, by delays in fixation, and by incorrect positioning on the substrate material. For these reasons, our endoscopists are asked to place the tissue immediately and directly into fixative. The histotechnologist then orients the biopsy in as nearly a vertical position as possible at the time of embedding. When this procedure is combined with the preparation of multiple sections, adequately-to-well oriented sections are usually found in one or more slides and at least as often as with the use of a substrate method.

In many laboratories, it is customary to cut and mount only one or two sections from each block. We regard this as an inadequate technique for study of IBD: We have repeatedly seen instances where placement of serial strips on two or more slides has significantly increased the amount of information obtained. In our laboratory, we make eight slides containing strips of serial sections from the biopsy specimens in each container submitted. Four slides (numbered 1, 3, 5, and 7) are stained with hematoxylin and eosin (H & E) and one (number 4) is stained with periodic acid-Schiff combined with Alcian blue (PAS-AB). The intervening slides are held in reserve for later staining if needed. Many laboratories are hesitant to follow a procedure such as this because of limitations in personnel and other resources, but we feel strongly that at least some additional slides and sections from each biopsy are essential.

NORMAL HISTOLOGY AND ARTEFACTUAL CHANGES

Normal Histology

A typical colo-rectal biopsy contains mucosa, muscularis mucosae, and a variable amount of submucosa. The mucosa shows evenly spaced, closely packed crypts, each of which has a tubular form of almost uniform width (Fig. 1), except in the neighborhood of lymphoid nodules. The bottoms of the crypts come close to

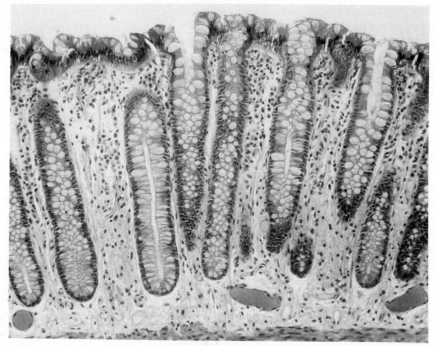

Fig. 1. Normal rectal biopsy. The crypts tend to be straight and parallel and do not branch. Variations in outline of crypts are due mainly to slight tilt from perpendicular of the plane of sectioning. Goblet cells are moderately prominent and the lamina propria shows normal cellularity. × 135.

the muscularis mucosae and line up evenly. The epithelium consists of goblet cells and undifferentiated cells containing little or no mucin. In a normal biopsy about 50% of the epithelial cells show mucin, although there are fewer goblet cells on the surface. There are scattered argyrophil cells and Paneth cells can sometimes be seen, especially in the right colon.

Lymphoid nodules may be biopsied either inadvertently or because they were noted grossly and regarded as a possible lesion. They are more common in preadolescents. Histologically, a lymphoid nodule consists of a collection of lymphocytes, sometimes with a germinal center, that lies in the mucosa and extends into the submucosa through an interruption in the muscularis mucosae (Fig. 2). Lymphoid nodules should not be confused with true chronic inflammation. Crypts adjacent to the lymphoid nodules are irregularly shaped and may show less mucin; there may also be additional epithelial mitoses in these crypts. These findings, too, must not be regarded as evidence of IBD.

The lamina propria in colo-rectal biopsies shows scattered lymphocytes and plasma cells and lesser numbers of histiocytes while the muscularis mucosae and submucosa contain only small numbers of mononuclear cells. Macrophages containing periodic acid-Schiff (PAS)-positive granules, termed muciphages (see below), are found so often in the rectal mucosa that they virtually represent a normal finding. Occasional eosinophils and basophils are also present.

CRUSH ARTEFACT

This is the most common form of artefact in colo-rectal biopsy material and results from the process of tissue removal. Some crush artefact during biopsy is unavoidable, but its severity varies depending on the condition of the biopsy instrument and the endoscopist's skill in obtaining tissue. The crush artefact may be due to compression at the point where the cutting edges meet and to a crimping effect that results when the amount of tissue taken exceeds the volume of the cup of the forceps (Fig. 3, *A* and *B*). Crush artefact can have a concentrating effect on the normal connective tissue, thereby giving the appearance of fibrosis. Severe crypt distortion which resembles that seen in long-standing IBD can also develop (Fig. 3, *C*). Another common manifestation of crush artefact is increased concentration of normal inflammatory cells that suggests true inflammation. Furthermore, the inflammatory cells are distorted, and irregularly shaped mononuclear cells may be misinterpreted as polymorphonuclear neutrophils (PMN) (Fig. 3, *D*).

ARTEFACT DUE TO ENEMAS AND LAXATIVES

These changes relate mainly to the enemas and other procedures which may be used to cleanse the large intestine before endoscopy. Patients are typically given 1 to 2 days of low residue diet followed by catharsis with castor oil or

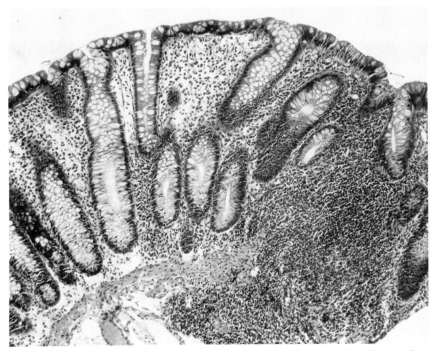

FIG. 2. Normal rectal biopsy containing a lymphoid nodule. The lymphoid cells extend into the submucosa , and the nearby crypts appear distorted. Lymphoid nodules should not be interpreted as due to inflammatory bowel disease. × 90.

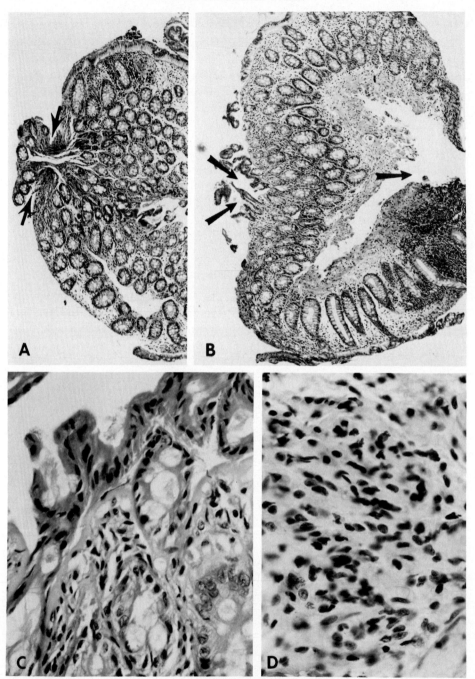

FIG. 3. Aspects of crush artefact. *A*, pinched tissue at base of biopsy (*arrows*) caused by dull blades on biopsy instrument. × 55. *B*, compressed, distorted mucosa in center of specimen resulting from crimping (*arrows*) during biopsy. × 55. *C*, detail from crimped area in *B*. There is damage to the epithelial cells and the lamina propria appears fibrotic. × 400. *D*, concentration and distortion of nuclei giving impression of inflammation. Some nuclei are so irregular in outline that they might be erroneously considered polymorphonuclear neutrophils. × 360.

magnesium citrate and a tapwater enema prior to colonoscopy. In our experience this causes no noticeable injury or inflammation to the mucosa although there may be a reduction in goblet cell mucin. Proctosigmoidoscopy is often performed in IBD without any prior cleansing procedure (the ideal method), and a single saline enema does not cause detectable injury.[50] On the other hand, a hypertonic, rapid-acting phosphate enema (Fleet type) or the suppository drug bisacodyl is sometimes used and they can lead to definite changes in the mucosa,[50] as can a soapsuds enema.[63] Experimental studies also suggest that Gastrografin used as a contrast material for x-ray studies can cause damage to the colonic mucosa.[43]

A Fleet enema or bisacodyl suppository can cause injury to the surface epithelium, reduced goblet cell mucin, edema, and acute inflammation[50] (Figs. 4, A and B). Numerous PMN may be seen marginating in capillaries and infiltrating the lamina propria and epithelium, especially at or near the mucosal surface. The time interval between the cleansing procedure and biopsy will obviously influence the type and degree of alterations noted. The changes are entirely reversible (Fig. 4, C).

It is self-evident that enema- or laxative-induced IBD might be mistaken for spontaneous IBD. Histologic features which help in recognizing acute IBD caused by patient preparation are: (1) uncharacteristically minimal or absent crypt inflammation when damage and inflammation in the surface epithelium and edema in the lamina propria are found to be prominent, (2) absence of

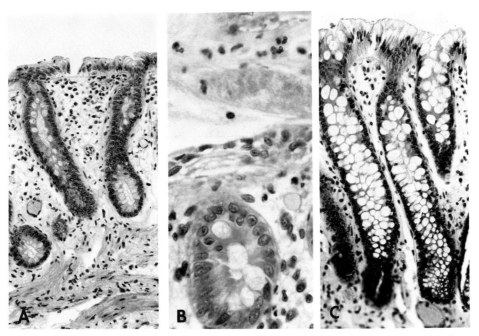

FIG. 4. *A*, rectal biopsy done about 30 minutes after administration of a hypertonic phosphate enema (Fleet). Mucosa is thinned and edematous and mucin in reduced. × 135. *B*, detail from *A* showing acute inflammation and damaged surface epithelium. × 525. *C*, repeat rectal biopsy done 5 days later without prior enema. The mucosa now appears normal. × 135.

associated increased chronic inflammation, and (3) absence of an associated increase in crypt mitoses (see below). These features result from the relatively short time interval between injury and biopsy, but they also presume a normal mucosa prior to administering the enema or suppository. Detecting enema- or laxative-induced IBD is much more difficult or even impossible when their effects have been superimposed on preexisting IBD.

BASIC HISTOLOGIC FINDINGS IN IBD: AN OVERVIEW

Most of the histopathologic findings in IBD are not specific for any one disease entity. For this reason the various histologic findings which must be dealt with when interpretating colo-rectal biopsies from patients with IBD are first described and discussed in a general way in this section and are listed in Table 1. Certain diseases are also mentioned, but the various specific forms of IBD are considered systematically in the section on differential diagnosis.

NONSPECIFIC ACUTE AND CHRONIC INFLAMMATION: GENERAL CHARACTERISTICS

Acute inflammation is easy to identify in a colo-rectal biopsy because even small numbers of PMN outside capillaries are an abnormal finding. Its character is similar for various forms of IBD.[25, 26] On the other hand, since mononuclear cells normally occur in the lamina propria, individual judgment can play an important role in determining chronic inflammation. While the proportion between acute and chronic inflammatory elements in IBD varies widely, in many situations where there is acute IBD the two forms of inflammation occur together almost from the onset. This holds true to some degree even for short-term, self-limited IBD due to infectious agents (*e. g.*, shigellosis) as well as for active stages of chronic IBD. Thus, while chronic inflammation may often be found in the absence of acute inflammation, acute inflammation without at least some evidence of chronic inflammation is not common in IBD, and minimal or

TABLE 1. COLO-RECTAL BIOPSY IN INFLAMMATORY BOWEL DISEASE (IBD): BASIC ASPECTS
OF HISTOPATHOLOGY

Nonspecific acute and chronic inflammation
  General characteristics
  Crypt abscesses
  Surface exudate and pseudomembrane formation
  Microscopic distribution (focal, patchy, and diffuse)
Granulomas and "granulomatous features"
Miscellaneous macrophage responses
  Muciphages
  Melanosis coli
  Barium granuloma
Epithelial alterations
  Mitotic increase
  Mucin decrease
  Injurious effects
  Atypia
Pseudopolyps (inflammatory polyps)
Necrosis, erosion, and ulceration
Active vs. inactive IBD

---

absent chronic inflammation should suggest the possibility of very acute injury such as that occurring after an enema or laxative. Reduction in chronic inflammatory cells, or absence of an expected increase, also occurs in patients on long-term, high dose treatment with corticosteroids or cytotoxic drugs (Fig. 5, *A*). Another abnormality is the absence of plasma cells in certain dysgammaglobulinemia syndromes that include a deficiency of IgA (Fig. 5, *B*).

Crypt Abscesses. Infiltration of the surface and crypt epithelium by PMN is a regularly noted aspect of acute inflammation in IBD (Fig. 6).[25] Crypt abscesses may be viewed as an outcome of heavy epithelial infiltration by PMN, representing the stage at which they reach the crypt lumen. Unfortunately, many physicians believe crypt abscesses are the hallmark of ulcerative colitis, *i. e.*, that their presence is diagnostic of that condition. This is entirely erroneous since crypt abscesses are a nonspecific observation which, while frequently

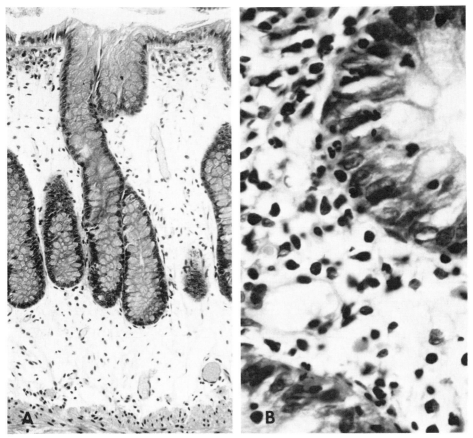

FIG. 5. Examples of altered lymphoid populations in rectal biopsies. *A*, overall reduction in lymphoid cells in a renal transplant patient receiving steroids and azothioprine. There is also some crypt distortion. × 160. *B*, absence of plasma cells in a patient with severely reduced serum IgA and IgM (common variable immune deficiency). Lymphocytes were present in normal or even increased numbers. Patient was a carrier of *Salmonella typhimurium*, and this is associated with acute inflammation in this biopsy. × 825.

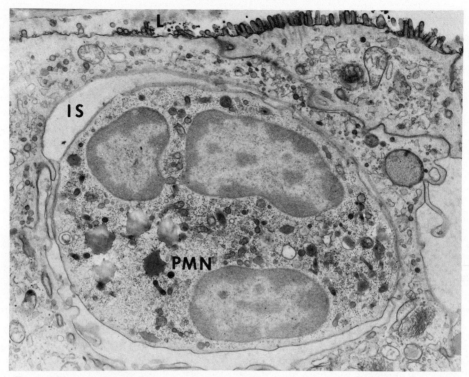

FIG. 6. Ultrastructural features of acute inflammation involving crypt epithelium. The patient had acute shigellosis. The crypt lumen (*L*) is at the top; a polymorphonuclear neutrophil (*PMN*) has migrated into the intercellular space (*IS*). Such *PMN* can eventually reach the crypt lumen to become part of a crypt abscess. × 6500. (Reproduced with permission from *The Johns Hopkins Medical Journal:* A. Gonzalez-Licea and J. H. Yardley: *Bulletin of the Johns Hopkins Hospital 118:* 444–461, 1966.

noted in ulcerative colitis (Fig. 13), are regularly seen in other forms of IBD (Figs. 15 and 18).

Surface Exudate and Pseudomembrane Formation. Exudate overlying the mucosa can be found in any form of IBD that shows acute inflammation (Figs. 4, 17*A*, 25, 29). The exudate typically consists of fibrin and variable amounts of mucin, PMN, and shed epithelial cells. Some cells may be necrotic. Surface exudate is often associated with breaks in the epithelial covering (erosions), presumably because they allow increased escape of protein and inflammatory cells.

Pseudomembrane is a descriptive term that most clearly applies to a grossly visible surface exudation that is thick, creamy, and adherent to the true membrane (the mucosa). Histologically, a pseudomembrane often shows much mucus, and the underlying mucosa is both heavily inflamed and is apt to demonstrate necrosis, mucus hypersecretion, and fibrin thrombi in capillaries. Ischemia can at times be important in the pathogenesis of necrosis and pseudo-membrane formation (see Chapter 2). The term pseudomembranous enterocolitis has been used by some authors to describe an entity which they believe is nosologically distinct.[10, 28, 49]

Inflammatory exudate overlying uninflamed mucosa is occasionally encountered. This discrepancy should be noted since it suggests that IBD is present in a more proximal area that may not have been viewed by the endoscopist.

Microscopic Distribution of Inflammation. Extension of inflammation below the mucosa is sometimes detectable in biopsy specimens, but depth of the inflammation is often impossible to assess realistically because of the small size and shallow depth of most biopsies.

The distribution pattern of inflammation in the lamina propria is characterizable as diffuse, focal, or patchy (Fig. 7). When diffuse, acute and chronic inflammation is more or less uniform everywhere in the mucosa. At the other extreme, inflammation is focal when it occurs in clearly identifiable areas in a mucosa that is not actively inflamed everywhere. Inflammation that is focal occasionally affects half or more of a biopsy specimen, but the foci are typically small and only a few crypts may be involved in the inflammation (Fig 17). The term patchy describes a distribution which lies somewhere between the extremes of diffuse and focal. Patchy inflammation shows variation in intensity from one area to the next, but at least some inflammation is seen almost everywhere. The various distribution patterns are not *per se* specific for any desease entity, but they can be very helpful in distinguishing between Crohn's disease and ulcerative colitis.

Granuloma and Granulomatous Features. In a colo-rectal biopsy the term granuloma refers to a well demarcated collection of epithelioid macrophages, usually with one or more multinucleated giant cells. Granulomas may be associated with other forms of inflammation or fibrosis or they may stand in pristine isolation. Eosinophils may be numerous in granulomas due to schistoso-

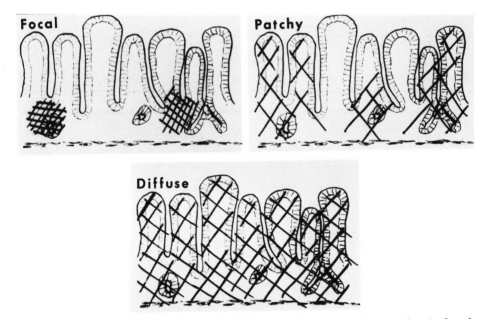

FIG. 7. The various distribution patterns which nonspecific inflammation can show in the colo-rectal mucosa are depicted schematically. Cross-hatching represents inflamed areas.

miasis. Granulomas may also show necrosis, caseous or otherwise, in some conditions, but they are typically hard (sarcoid-like) in Crohn's disease. Special stains for organisms should be done if necrosis is present, if findings in the conventional H & E histologic preparation suggest a causative agent, or if the clinical picture warrants it. On the other hand, because of a uniformily negative experience, we do not routinely perform stains for causative agents on noncaseous granulomatous lesions from patients who are believed to have Crohn's disease.

Misdiagnosis of a lymphoid germinal center as a granuloma ordinarily traps only the novice, but all should be alert to the possibility. Another finding that can imitate a granuloma is a collection of crypt epithelial cells that has been shaved off in the plane of sectioning. The real nature of such a finding is easily verified in adjacent sections.

While well delineated granulomas, especially those containing giant cells, are relatively easy to recognize, there are also borderline forms of granulomatous inflammation which should be searched for. These consist of relatively discrete areas of nonspecific inflammation which are found to contain cells with fairly large vesicular nuclei of the type noted in epithelioid macrophages. When this finding is clearly present, we append the term granulomatous features to our description of the inflammation.

Miscellaneous Macrophage Responses. Macrophages with mucinous cytoplasmic contents are present in the lamina propria of up to 50% of all rectal biopsies. They are less common in the colon. Only a scattering of these cells, termed muciphages by Azzopardi,[2] are usually found, but they may be numerous, occurring throughout the mucosa and sometimes in the submucosa. A typical location for muciphages is the area just under the surface epithelium. The cytoplasm is foamy in H & E-stained sections. With PAS-AB staining discrete intracytoplasmic granules are seen (Fig. 8). Muciphages occur with about equal frequency in normal individuals and in patients with IBD.[27] Their chief importance lies in their ability to trap the unwary into a misdiagnosis. Muciphages will occasionally be regarded as epithelioid macrophages and hence as evidence for Crohn's disease or some other granulomatous entity. An even more common error is to assume, because the macrophages are PAS-positive, that the patient may have Whipple's disease.

Pigmented macrophages in melanosis coli are easily recognized by their golden brown cytoplasmic lipofuscin; it can also be PAS-positive. Except for the rare patient with chronic inorganic mercury poisoning or with so-called cathartic colon,[56] melanosis coli does not relate in any particular way to IBD.

Barium sulphate occasionally enters the mucosa and submucosa during a barium enema and the insoluble crystals are phagocytosed by macrophages. These then collect as barium granulomas. The barium sulphate crystals have a characteristic light green color, do not polarize, and are PAS-negative. Staining with sodium rhodizonate can be used to identify the barium.[61]

Epithelial Alterations. Epithelial cells are highly sensitive to injurious agents and tend to respond similarly in all forms of IBD. In addition to visible evidence of cell injury, there are two early changes in the epithelium which can signal active inflammatory bowel disease: 1) increased numbers of mitotic figures in the epithelial cells of the crypts, and 2) reduced epithelial mucin (Fig. 9). An

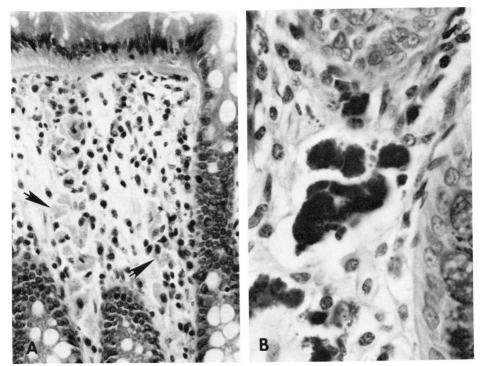

Fig. 8. *A*, Muciphages in the lamina propria are seen as clusters (*arrows*) of cells having abundant, pale cytoplasm. Hematoxylin and eosin, × 300. *B*, the muciphages are filled with granules which stain heavily for neutral and acid mucopolysaccharides. Combined PAS-AB stain. × 750.

increased number of mitotic figures reflects heightened cell turnover in response to injury. Approximately one mitotic figure in every 2 to 3 crypts is normally seen in sectioned material, and a definite increase can be regarded as present when one or more mitotic figures are found in nearly every crypt. Reduced mucin content presumably comes about from increased stimulation to its secretion, perhaps combined with lessened time for synthesis as a result of the shorter epithelial life span. Crypts showing reduced epithelial mucin tend to correspond in distribution to the inflammatory process (Fig. 21).

Severity of epithelial injury increases in parallel with increasingly severe and prolonged IBD. The cells may become flattened and condensed-looking and detached from the basement membrane. Some crypts may eventually be destroyed so that crypt-free gaps appear in the mucosa, while crypts that survive become misshapened and may show branching that persists after subsidence of the active disease (Fig. 10).

Nuclear changes which give the epithelial cells an immature, and even atypical (dysplastic) appearance, develop when inflammation is intense. The atypia is most severe in the crypt bases, diminishing progressively towards the surface, a finding that helps to distinguish it from precancerous changes (see Chapter 8). Atypia is also marked in epithelium which is actively regenerating over ulcers, and it may be a prominent finding in radiation injury (Fig. 28).

Pseudopolyps (Inflammatory Polyps). Any discrete lesion attached to the

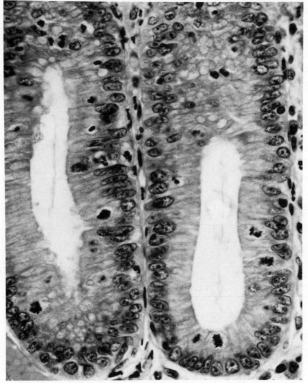

Fɪɢ. 9. Increased numbers of mitotic figures in epithelial cells and reduced epithelial mucin in otherwise relatively mild inflammatory bowel disease (ulcerative colitis). × 525.

mucosa, no matter what its pathogenesis, can be rightfully termed a polyp, and for this reason pseudopolyps are definitely not pseudo. (Perhaps the word was originally coined to indicate that the polyps are false in the sense that they are non-neoplastic). Despite the inherent inaccuracy, we use this well established term for this characteristic finding in IBD as it is unambiguous and makes no assumptions about pathogenesis.

Pseudopolyps vary in appearance and makeup histologically, but there are two basic components: 1) variable amounts of inflamed granulation tissue, and 2) markedly distorted crypts which may appear as bizarre, hyperplastic, branching, and often inflamed glands that may be dilated or cystic (Fig. 11). Thus pseudopolyps typically show loss of organization as mucosa, *i. e.*, the usual pattern of crypts lined up in a regular fashion over the muscularis mucosae disappears. The epithelial cells of a pseudopolyp are often tall, hyperplastic, and mucin-containing.

While a mixture of the epithelial and inflammatory components is most common,[42] in some pseudopolyps the irregular glandular structures predominate while others consist almost solely of inflamed granulation tissue with little or no epithelial elements. The contrast with adjacent mucosa that has not been transformed into pseudopolyps may be striking.

Ulceration is often found in the vicinity of pseudopolyps, suggesting that they

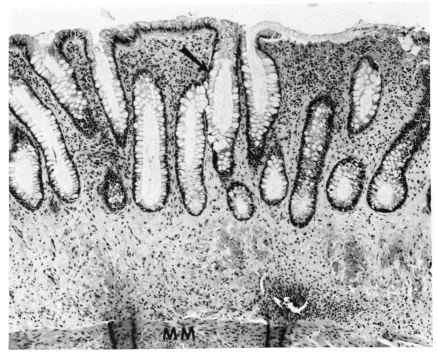

Fig. 10. An example of inactive inflammatory bowel disease (IBD) with moderately severe crypt distortion. The crypts are irregular in shape, and their orientation is generally nonparallel. One crypt shows branching (*arrow*). Others are bulbous at their bases. Also, the space between crypts and the muscularis mucosae (*MM*) is widened and contains fibrous tissue. The abundant mucin and the fact that no acute inflammation was seen also indicated that the IBD was inactive. × 85.

are an exaggerated, disordered healing response of the mucosa between ulcers.[59] After subsidence of inflammation the pseudopolyps may be retained as thin, elongated tags of mucosa.

Pseudopolyps are most commonly noted in ulcerative colitis, but can be seen in any form of chronic IBD. They may be single or multiple and sometimes become very large.[81] In schistosomiasis and histoplasmosis the causative agent is prominently displayed in the pseudopolyps.

The small size of a colo-rectal biopsy specimen may preclude definite identification of a pseudopolyp. However, a biopsy that consists mainly or entirely of granulation tissue, often with polypoid outline, or one that shows clumps of highly irregular, disoriented and hyperplastic glands that are inflamed, is highly suggestive (Fig. 11). Correlation with endoscopic findings is frequently confirmatory. The lack of a demonstrable direct relationship between pseudopolyps and precancerous changes is discussed in Chapter 8.

Erosion, Ulceration, and Necrosis. Erosion is defined as discrete loss of musoca that does not extend entirely through the mucosa. Ulceration is any deeper lesion. Limitations imposed by the small size of biopsy specimens can obviously make it difficult to arrive at a distinction between the two. One should assume, however, that there is erosion or ulceration in specimens that demon-

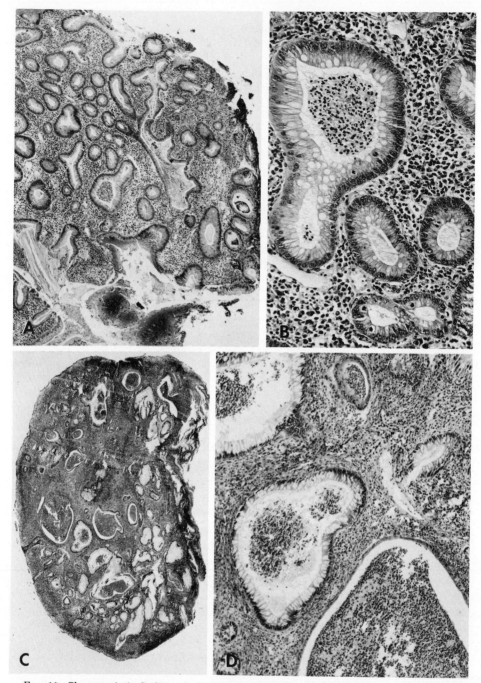

FIG. 11. Characteristic findings in biopsy specimens from pseudopolyps. *A*, an irregularly shaped tissue fragment containing distorted, inflamed glands rather than recognizable crypts. This pattern in a biopsy suggests pseudopolyp formation even when they were not described endoscopically. × 35. *B*, detail from *A* showing irregular outline of glands, inflammation, and hyperplastic epithelium. × 175. *C*, small pseudopolyp removed in its entirety. × 16. *D*, detail from *C* showing prominent fibrosis in addition to other changes. × 80.

strate inflamed granulation tissue and necrotic debris, especially in biopsies where no recognizable mucosa is found and if smooth muscle and connective tissue are present.

Some necrosis, as judged by the usual criteria for cell death, may be seen in any type of IBD. Small areas of necrosis confined to the mucosa are much more common than is extensive or total necrosis of the type that occurs in widespread ischemia. Necrosis is usually so intimately associated with erosion or ulceration that determining whether it preceded or followed the loss of mucosa is not possible.

Active vs. Inactive IBD. Acute inflammation is the principal finding that defines activity of IBD. Other changes associated with active IBD – chronic inflammation, loss of epithelial mucin, increased numbers of mitotic figures in epithelial cells, necrosis, ulceration, granulomas, etc. – can be helpful but are less reliable or are present too inconstantly. In ulcerative colitis, a biopsy is often specifically performed to assess disease activity since histologic evidence of inflammation in ulcerative colitis is a more sensitive guage of activity than clinical or endoscopic findings.[14, 48, 83] Colo-rectal biopsy is less valuable for following activity in patients with Crohn's disease because of the irregular distribution of changes.

When IBD becomes quiescent or heals, the mucosa is often left in a permanently altered state and will show characteristic histologic changes (Fig. 10) even, at times, when the bowel was thought to be normal by endoscopy. The principal findings in inactive IBD are: (1) scarring and basement membrane thickening, (2) crypt distortion, (3) mucosal thinning (atrophy) and loss of crypts, and (4) widening of the space between crypt bases and the muscularis mucosae. In our experience the most reliable single feature for diagnosing healed or inactive IBD is the branched crypt, this abnormality being difficult to account for by any mechanism other than regeneration after injury.

Inactive IBD is, in general, qualitatively independent of the patient's original disease type. Severity and distribution of scarring, atrophy, and crypt distortion tend to correlate, however, with the intensity, duration, and distribution of the IBD when it was active. The changes will be negligible following an acute, self-limited episode of infectious colitis, and they will be most marked after severe, long-standing IBD as in ulcerative colitis. It is self-evident that minor degrees of fibrosis and crypt distortion should not be overinterpreted as evidence for healed or inactive IBD, particularly when crush artefact may be present.

DIFFERENTIAL DIAGNOSIS

General Approach. Significant diagnostic limitations are set by the small size of colo-rectal biopsies and by the fact that in the last analysis most histologic changes in IBD are nonspecific. Yet it is often possible to arrive at a useful statement about a patient's condition by examining the biopsy specimens systematically and by considering them in the light of other known facts about the patient. Our general procedure with colo-rectal biopsy specimens in IBD can be summarized as follows: (1) If histologic evidence of either active or inactive IBD is present, infectious agents or other features that might suggest a specific diagnosis are searched for. (2) Histologic findings are compared with endoscopic and clinical observations and with previous histologic material. (3) If all facts are most consistent with chronic idiopathic IBD, further characterization is attempted *i. e.*, as ulcerative colitis or Crohn's disease.

The merging of histologic, endoscopic, and clinical findings is enhanced by an efficient method for transmitting information from the endoscopist to the pathologist. A specially designed requisition form (Fig. 12) is of great assistance, its key feature being a diagram on which lesions and biopsy sites can be quickly and accurately noted.

While the pathologist's written diagnostic statement (sign-out) should always be as specific as possible, the available facts often limit him or her to a description of the findings and to an indication that IBD of unknown type is present. An example of such a limited sign-out is: "Rectum (biopsy): Diffuse acute and chronic inflammation with crypt distortion and increased epithelial mitotic figures consistent with inflammatory bowel disease, type indeterminant." It is essential that the pathologist not be overly swayed by clinical impressions and thereby mislead the clinician into believing a definitive histologic diagnosis has been reached when it has not. On the other hand, it is also important to discuss differential possibilities and to indicate consistency or inconsistency of the pathologic findings with a clinical judgment. This is often best done in an additional note which is kept separate from the sign-out statement. For instance, if the gastroenterologist feels the patient has ulcerative colitis, and if the findings in the biopsy are those expected in that disease, we say so in a note. On the other hand, when the IBD is of recent onset the possibility of a self-limited disorder, perhaps of infectious origin, will be stressed. Thus the histologic findings are always considered in the context of their larger meaning to the patient in the belief that pathologists should participate actively in the total diagnostic process.

Table 2 lists the principal disease entities that comprise IBD. The table also serves as an outline for the remainder of this section. The key pathologic findings in colo-rectal biopsies from each of the listed disorders will be discussed along with pertinent clinical and pathogenetic observations.

Chronic Idiopathic IBD. A large proportion of all biopsies in IBD are obtained from patients with either ulcerative colitis or Crohn's disease, and deciding between these two entities is often a major objective. Pathologic findings in ulcerative colitis and Crohn's disease from the standpoint of the entire specimen have been frequently described and are well covered in Chapter 1. This discussion will, therefore, deal primarily with histopathologic features which are pertinent to the interpretation of colo-rectal biopsies.

The important endoscopic correlations and microscopic findings in active ulcerative colitis and Crohn's disease are summarized in Table 3.

While the endoscopist must describe and record gross findings in idiopathic IBD prior to biopsy, the pathologist still plays an important role in their final interpretation by noting the distribution of histopathologic observations in biopsies from several areas. In this way the presence of a diffuse lesion with distal predominance favoring ulcerative colitis might be verified in one patient while in another patient the histologic observations may indicate right-sided predominance, skip areas, or relative rectal sparing, findings which weren't

ENDOSCOPIC FINDINGS (Use diagram to show location of lesion(s) and biopsy sites, etc.)

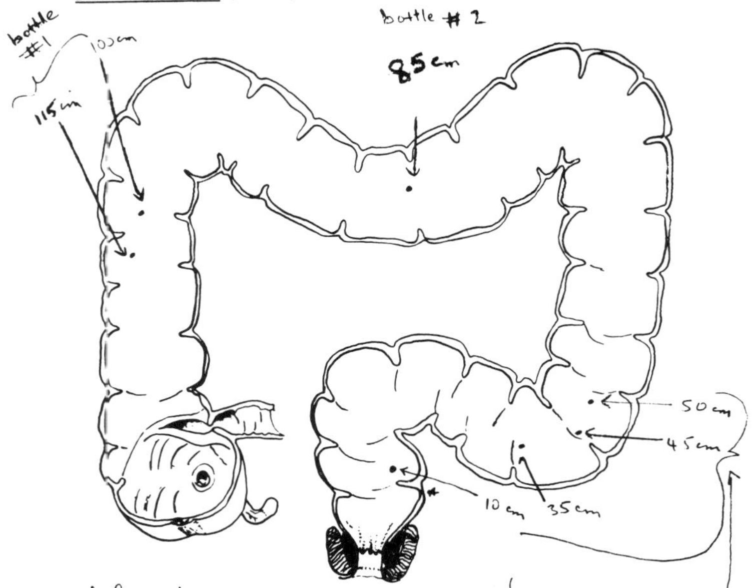

bottle #2

85 cm

bottle #1

(100 cm)

(115 cm)

10 cm 35 cm

45 cm

50 cm

bottle #3

~35 cm in rectum up to

mild friability, opacity, + loss of submucosal vessels in rectum + sigmoid up to ~35 cm

ENDOSCOPIC DIAGNOSES:

(1) ulcerative colitis

(2) disease confined to rectum and sigmoid

(3) minimal activity at present

Signature _____ M.D.

BACK

Surgical Pathology No. _____

The Johns Hopkins Hospital
Recto-Colonic Biopsy Requisition and Data Sheet

Pt's Name _____

Age 40   Race W   Sex F   Hist. # _____   Date __/__/__   Ward or Clinic ACops

Operator _____

APPROVED BY
T. P1

Prior Operations or Biopsies: Yes __ No __
JHH ___, Elsewhere (where?) _____
Particulars, if known:

Major Clinical Findings (Hx, P.E., Lab. etc.):

15 year history of ulcerative proctitis, in remission clinically for several months. Patient concerned about chance of developing.

Reasons for Endoscopy and Biopsy:

Assess activity of her U.C. + R/o premalignant or malignant changes.

- - - - - - - Space Below for Lab Use Only - - - - - - - - - (See Reverse Side)

Specimen(s) Received: _____

1. Rectal Bx at 115 & 109 cm - 3 pc largest meas 0.5x0.4x0.2 cm
2. Rectal Bx " 85 cm - 1pc meas 0.4x0.2 cm
3. Rectal Bx " 50, + 3; 8cm 35 & 10 cm 4pc largest meas 0.4x0.2x0.2 cm

FRONT

FIG. 12. Requisition form used at the The Johns Hopkins Hospital for colonoscopic biopsies. Information on an actual patient is shown (personal identifications obscured).

TABLE 2. CLASSIFICATION OF INFLAMMATORY BOWEL DISEASE (IBD)

Idiopathic IBD
  Ulcerative colitis and proctitis
  Crohn's disease
Bacterial IBD
  Dysenteric (*Shigella, Salmonella,* pathogenic *Escherichia coli, etc.*)
  Gonococcal proctitis
  Tuberculous
  Whipple's disease
Parasitic IBD
  Amebiasis
  Balantidiasis
  Schistosomiasis
  Cryptosporidiosis
Viral IBD
  Lymphogranuloma venereum
  Cytomegalovirus
Fungal IBD
  Histoplasmosis
Drug, chemical and foodstuff-related IBD
  Antibiotic-related
  Cytotoxic drugs (5-FU)-related
  Heavy metal-related
  Milk protein allergy
Irradiation-induced IBD
  Acute irradiation colitis
  Post-irradiation colitis
IBD of intrinsic origin
  Ischemic colitis
  Solitary ulcer syndrome
  Diverticulitis
  Obstruction-related
Pseudomembranous enterocolitis

even necessarily clear-cut endoscopically, but which support Crohn's disease.[21] To arrive at such distinctions the pathologist must always accurately record histologic findings in a way that can be correlated with the endoscopic observations.

Rectal involvement in Crohn's disease requires special comment. Some physicians believe that rectal sparing must be both grossly and histologically complete to be consistent with that disorder. Instead, the rectum may only appear grossly to be less inflamed as compared to more proximal large intestine. At the same time there may be much more inflammation than was expected clinically because inflammation in Crohn's disease is often grossly and histologically focal. For the same reason inflammation may be intense in one specimen and much reduced or even absent in another. The irregular distribution, which is an important distinguishing characteristic of Crohn's disease, is most reliably demonstrated by sampling both maximally and minimally involved mucosa.

While ulcerative colitis typically shows little or no variation within the confines of the rectum or short colonic segments, Price (Chapter 1) has commented on the fact that relative rectal sparing may be found in a few patients with ulcerative colitis, perhaps because of treatment with steroid suppositories.

We have also seen misleading "skip lesions" in ulcerative colitis which resulted from severe pseudopolyposis that ended sharply just above the rectum.

When considering the character of the inflammaton in idiopathic IBD, it is noteworthy that granulomas are not found in most biopsy specimens from patients with Crohn's disease. One group of investigators saw them 19% of the time[15] and we found granulomas in only four of 32 specimens (12%) in the study of focal lesions described below. Granulomas having several appearances in rectal biopsy specimens from Crohn's disease are illustrated in Fig. 13. Detection of even one multinucleated giant cell, usually of the Langhan's type, provides valuable confirmatory evidence of a granuloma, especially when macrophages are sparse or form an ill-defined collection.

Granulomatous features in nonspecific inflammation are not unheard of in patients who have ulcerative colitis (Table 3), especially, perhaps, when the disease process is relatively quiescent. Yet we find that granulomatous features (Fig. 14) provide useful supportive evidence of Crohn's disease since they are distinctly more common and prominent in that entity. Cook and Dixon[8] also found such changes, which they termed "numerous histiocytes" and "epithelioid cell follicles", to be more frequent in Crohn's disease.

Ordinary nonspecific acute and chronic inflammation is, of course, the major form taken by the inflammatory process in both ulcerative colitis and Crohn's disease. As was emphasized previously, crypt abscesses do not reliably help in choosing between ulcerative colitis and Crohn's disease. Even though they occur more often in Crohn's disease, we find that ulceration, erosion, and submucosal extension of inflammation are not consistently trustworthy distinguishing features in colo-rectal biopsies. It is also clear that biopsies from ulcerative colitis can show some submucosal inflammation, usually in severe cases (see Chapter 1). Normal lymphoid nodules extending into the submucosa can further complicate interpretation of this feature.

Not so widely recognized is the fact that the distribution of nonspecific inflammation within the lamina propria can often be of great value in deciding whether idiopathic IBD is due to ulcerative colitis or to Crohn's disease. While the presence of diffuse or patchy inflammation (Figs. 15 and 16) is not helpful in making the diagnostic distinction, when there is clear-cut focal nonspecific inflammation, most characteristically as a lesion within one biopsy (Fig. 17) but also as variation in amount of inflammation in contiguous biopsies, Crohn's disease is strongly favored over ulcerative colitis.

We verified this point more objectively by examining the distribution of nonspecific inflammation in rectal biopsies from 30 patients who had active ulcerative colitis, Crohn's disease, ulcerative proctitis, or idiopathic IBD of indeterminate type. Patient selection was random except that those with ulcerative colitis were included only when there was histologically active disease. (Biopsies showing inactive ulcerative colitis were usually obtained by the endoscopist to assess disease activity. Hence frequency of inactive disease had no special significance). Clinical, radiologic, and pathologic information was used to determine the final patient classification. All histologic slides from 54 biopsies were coded and examined by two observers. Histologic criteria for determining focal, patchy, or diffuse distribution were those described under "Basic Histologic Findings."

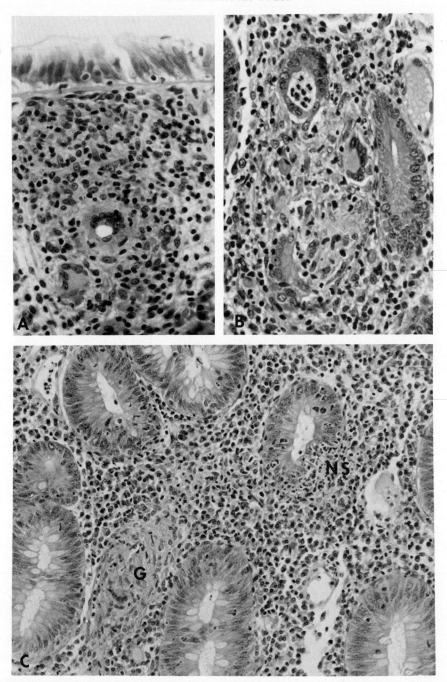

FIG. 13. Some examples of granulomas in Crohn's disease. *A*, a sarcoid-like granuloma containing giant cells, epithelioid macrophages, and lymphocytes. No polymorphonuclear neutrophils are seen here. (One giant cell contains an artefactual vacuole.) × 325. *B*, a granuloma with related acute inflammation and severe damage to crypts and with crypt abscess formation is noted. × 325. *C*, a granuloma (*G*) is seen near a separate focus of nonspecific acute and chronic inflammation (*NS*). × 110.

TABLE 3. ULCERATIVE COLITIS (UC) VS. CROHN'S DISEASE OF THE COLON (CD): FREQUENCY OF PATHOLOGIC FINDINGS BY COLO-RECTAL BIOPSY IN ACTIVE DISEASE

	UC	CD
Endoscopic correlations		
Total proctocolitis	+++	+
Distal predominance	++++	+
Right colon predominance	0	+++
Rectal sparing (relative)	+	+++
Skip areas	0	+++
Punctate lesions	0	++
Microscopic character of inflammation		
Granulomas	0	+
Nonspecific with granulomatous features	+	++
Nonspecific acute & chronic	++++	+++
Microscopic distribution of nonspecific inflammation		
Crypt abscesses	++++	++
Associated ulceration or erosion	+	+ or ++
Submucosal extension (any)	++	+++
Diffuse (lamina propria)	++++	++
Patchy (lamina propria)	++	++
Focal (lamina propria)	0	++

Key for frequency (estimated) of findings in active idiopathic IBD: 0 = never seen or very rare, + = uncommon (<20%), ++ = fairly common (20–50%), +++ = common (50–80%), ++++ = very common (>80%).

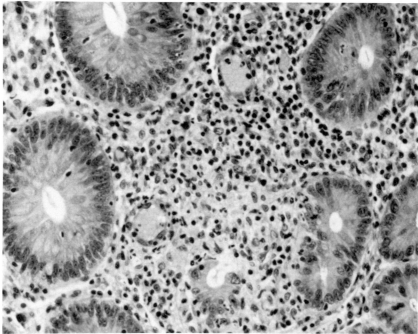

FIG. 14. Non-specific inflammation with "granulomatous features" in another area from biopsy shown in Fig. 13, *B*. Macrophages are moderately prominent and show some tendency to aggregate, but there are no giant cells. There are damaged crypts and dilated capillaries. When noted in idiopathic inflammatory bowel disease, granulomatous features increase the possibility of Crohn's disease although the finding has much less specificity than a full-blown granuloma. × 325.

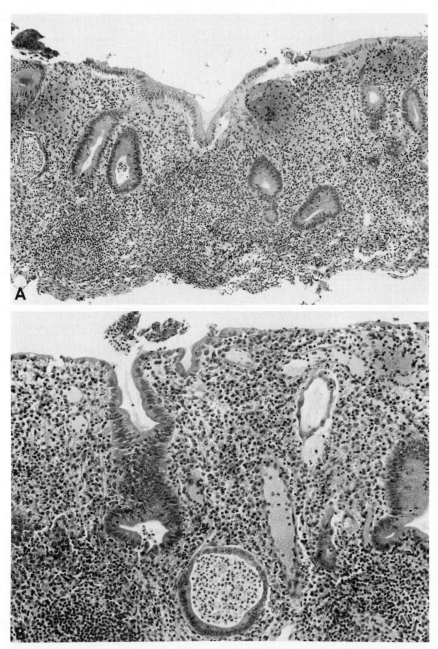

Fig. 15. Diffuse inflammation in ulcerative colitis. *A*, the inflammation is severe and is of similar intensity everywhere. Some crypts have been destroyed and remaining crypts show distortion and presence of abscesses. Lymphoid nodules are also increased in number. This is at times a prominent feature in active ulcerative colitis. × 90. *B*, same specimen. The inflammatory reaction is composed predominently of lymphocytes, plasma cells, and polymorphologic neutrophils. A crypt abscess is demonstrated. The surface epithelium is damaged but intact. × 150.

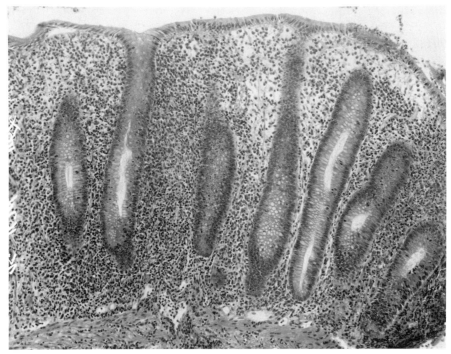

FIG. 16. An example of inflammation that is more patchy in ulcerative colitis. Relative sparing from inflammation is seen in some areas. × 150.

The results (Table 4) strongly favored association of focal inflammation with Crohn's disease. While focal inflammation was not seen in any of the 14 biopsy specimens from patients with active ulcerative colitis, it occurred in 10 of 23 showing active inflammatory disease from patients with Crohn's disease. Another nine biopsy specimens showed no active inflammatory lesion.

It is important to stress that inflammation in Crohn's disease, especially when it is focal, can be seen in rectal biopsy specimens when the disorder is thought clinically to be limited to the small intestine or to the small intestine and cecum, as well as in those with Crohn's disease of the more distal colon and rectum (Table 4). Because of this finding, which has been noted by others,[15, 21] rectal biopsy can be a useful procedure in all patients with suspected Crohn's disease, including those who show no radiologic or endoscopic disease in the distal colon and rectum.

The frequent occurrence of focal inflammation in Crohn's disease as compared to ulcerative colitis has been described previously.[16, 26, 35] In an elegant computerized study, focal inflammatory lesions in rectal biopsy specimens were observed preferentially in Crohn's disease at a highly significant level ($P <$ 0.001).[35] Many observers also emphasize the related focal or irregular reduction in goblet cell mucin which is seen in Crohn's disease.[11, 31, 56, 67] In our experience, however, disparities in loss of mucin from goblet cells are more useful for establishing the diagnosis of Crohn's disease in resected specimens than in colo-rectal biopsy specimens because of their limited size.

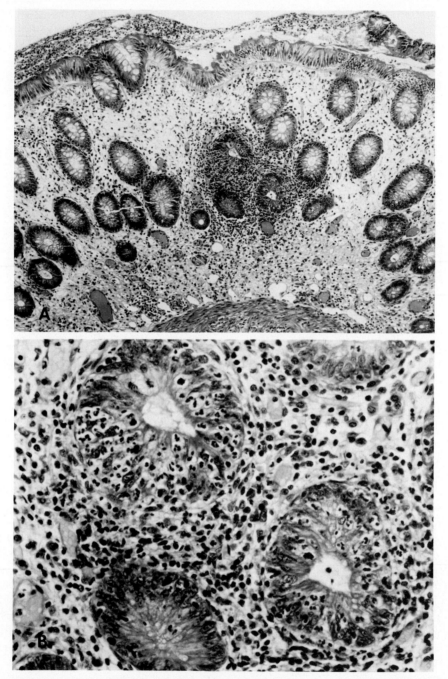

FIG. 17. Focal nonspecific inflammation in Crohn's disease. *A*, there is a well delineated focus of inflammation with surrounding uninflamed mucosa. Inflammatory exudate is present on the surface. × 90. *B*, lymphocytes and polymorphonuclear neutrophils predominate in the inflammatory focus seen in *A*. Crypts are markedly inflamed and damaged. × 350.

TABLE 4. RECTAL BIOPSIES IN ULCERATIVE COLITIS AND CROHN'S DISEASE

Disease (Number of patients)	Distribution of nonspecific acute and chronic inflammation in mucosa[a]			
	Focal	Patchy	Diffuse	Absent
Ulcerative colitis (11)	0	2	12	0[b]
Crohn's disease[c]				
All Crohn's (15)	10	4	9	9
S.I.[d] or S.I. + cecum (7)	2	0	0	5
S.I. + colon distal to cecum (5)	2	3	2	0
Colon only (3)	6	1	7	4
Ulcerative proctitis (1)	0	1	1	0
Indeterminate IBD[e] (3)	2	0	4	4

[a] Numbers of biopsy specimens are indicated.
[b] Biopsy specimens showing only inactive disease not used (see text).
[c] Subdivided by clinically determined distribution of disease.
[d] S.I. = small intestine.
[e] IBD = inflammatory bowel disease.

Focal nonspecific lesions, nonspecific inflammation with granulomatous features, and true granulomas may represent different degrees or stages of related pathologic processes in Crohn's disease. Indeed, we have seen colo-rectal biopsy specimens where focal, nonspecific inflammatory lesions merged with true granulomas (Fig. 13, *C*).

It is evident that histologic findings offer fewer choices for diagnosis of ulcerative colitis than they do for recognizing Crohn's disease (Table 3). Diagnosis of ulcerative colitis relies much more, therefore, on analysis of the total clinical picture. The pathologist must carefully avoid exaggerating the evidence for one or another form of chronic idiopathic colitis, accepting the fact that some cases must be described as indeterminant as to type of colitis.

Ulcerative proctitis is a nonspecific acute and chronic inflammation of the rectum which is histologically indistinguishable from ulcerative colitis. Diagnosis of ulcerative proctitis depends on combining clinical findings, which are those of a less severe illness, with endoscopic demonstration that the inflammatory process is limited to the rectum. Persuasive arguments can be made that ulcerative proctitis is a nosologically distinct entity,[18] but many observers feel that it is only a milder, less extensive version of ulcerative colitis. This view is supported by colonoscopic studies which indicate that patients with ulcerative proctitis can show inflammation, albeit mild, in the proximal colon.[74]

Bacterial IBD. The inflammatory changes in bacterial dysentery due to *Shigella* vary widely in severity.[1] Because of lower mortality, less is known about colitis in human beings caused by the nontyphoid *salmonellae* and other pathogenic gram negative rods, but experimental studies[37] suggest that the lesion is qualitatively similar to that seen in shigellosis.

Biopsy specimens in shigellosis typically show nonspecific acute inflammation which is sometimes patchy. Chronic inflammation may be mild or absent.[55] Surface exudate is often prominent and in severe cases it is seen as a thick, creamy pseudomembrane. Surface epithelial cells are frequently damaged and infiltrated by PMN, and mucin content is markedly reduced.[70] Crypt abscesses are not common, but they can occur (Fig. 18). It is generally accepted that the causative organism must invade the mucosa to establish disease (see Chapter 3). Invading organisms can be demonstrated in the lamina propria by using fluorescent antibody,[19, 37] but this is primarily an experimental method. Gram staining of biopsy specimens usually achieves no practical purpose since the bacteria are often difficult to detect in this way, and nonpathogenic secondary invaders from the lumen also occur. The key step in diagnosis of bacterial dysentery remains, therefore, isolation of the agent by culture.

It is obviously essential that patients who are only suffering from an acute, self-limited infectious enterocolitis not be labeled as having idiopathic IBD. A chronic colitis rarely develops following an episode of shigellosis, but this is an ill-defined outcome. On the other hand, we have seen a chronic carrier state for *Salmonella typhimurium* following an episode of food poisoning in a patient with deficient local immunity. There was persistent acute inflammation in addition to the absence of plasma cells (Fig. 5, *B*).

Gonococcal proctitis is another acute exudative nonspecific inflammatory condition. It develops by genito-anal spread in females and results from anal intercourse in males.[39] Demonstration of numerous gram negative diplococci in the exudate leads to a presumptive diagnosis, but as in the bacterial dysenteries, definitive diagnosis depends on culture of the organisms.

Although the distal ileum is the most frequent site of intestinal tuberculosis,

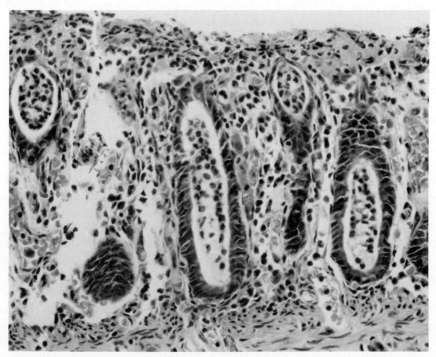

FIG. 18. Rectal biopsy in severe shigellosis. There is marked acute inflammation with crypt abscesses, loss of goblet cell mucin, and epithelial damage. × 80.

tuberculosis of the colon and rectum were at one time also considered fairly common.[60] It is now a rare disorder, and we have not seen a case in our own biopsy material. Findings which should suggest tuberculosis are: (1) numerous and/or large granulomas, (2) presence of caseation, (3) demonstration of acid-fast bacilli. It is likely, of course, that some patients who in the past were thought to have colo-rectal tuberculosis actually had Crohn' disease since the two entities share many features.

Whipple's disease is a rare bacterial infection which is usually centered in the small intestine;[32] the causative organism remains unidentified. PAS-positive macrophages appear in many organs in Whipple's disease including the rectum.[27] The rectum has also looked grossly inflamed in at least one patient[84] even though acute inflammation was not present. The recurring problem for pathologists is to distinguish between the commonly seen PAS and Alcian blue-positive muciphages and the PAS-stained macrophages which occur in the very rare case of Whipple's disease that they encounter. Numerous PAS-positive macrophages in a rectal biopsy from a patient with unexplained diarrheal illness should certainly raise at least some suspicion of Whipple's disease. And if the macrophages are Alcian blue-negative, the intracytoplasmic inclusions are small (Fig. 19), or rod-shaped extracellular objects consistent with small organisms are

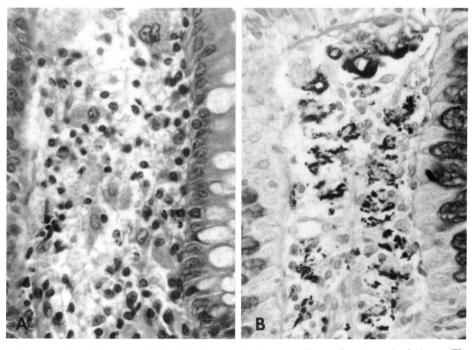

FIG. 19. Rectal biopsy in Whipple's disease. *A*, hematoxylin- and eosin-stained tissue. The lamina propria shows foamy macrophages that are not distinguishable from muciphages. × 480. *B*, same tissue stained by both the PAS and Alcian blue methods. The macrophages were found to contain only PAS positive granules and these tend to be smaller than muciphage granules (compare with Fig. 8). While these findings can suggest Whipple's disease, presence of Alcian blue-positive granules cannot rule out the diagnosis (see Fig. 20). × 480.

noted, then the suspicion should be greater. Alcian blue-stained macrophages occur also, however, in Whipple's disease of the rectum (Fig. 20). Definitive determination of whether or not a patient has Whipple's disease depends, therefore, on jejunal biopsy.[27]

Parasitic IBD. Amebiasis occurs most commonly as an ulcerative disease of the cecum and right colon. It can, however, present as a chronic or acute form of IBD involving the left colon and rectum, often with only small or no grossly visible ulcerations.[3, 24, 64] This fact is not always appreciated by clinicians and pathologists, especially in the western countries where idiopathic IBD predominates over amebic and other infectious forms of IBD, and it can be a serious matter. Overlooking the diagnosis of amebic colitis not only deprives the patient of a likely cure, but there is also the risk that his condition will be worsened if corticosteroids are given.[3] For this reason all patients with chronic IBD should initially have a well conducted examination of their stools for trophozoites and a test of their serum for antibodies to amebae.

The mucosa in amebiasis can show all degrees of involvement from slight nonspecific inflammatory changes through erosion to frank ulceration.[65, 66] The inflammation may be diffuse or focal with micro-ulcers (erosions); localized loss of mucin is also characteristic (Fig. 21).[65, 66] Biopsy is not the preferred method

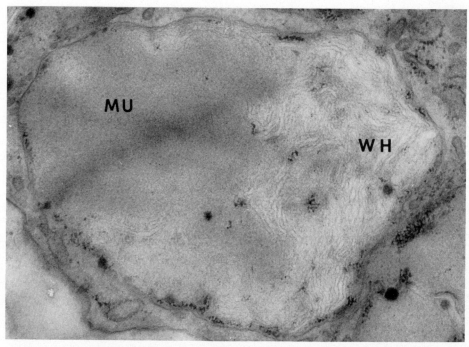

FIG. 20. Electron micrograph of a macrophage in a rectal biopsy from Whipple's disease. An amorphous substance like that found in muciphages (*MU*) and typical membranous material of Whipple's disease (*WH*) are present in a single membrane-bounded granule. Such findings account well for occurrence at times of staining for muciphage and Whipple type inclusions in the same rectal macrophage. × 64,800. (Reproduced with permission from : A. Gonzalez-Licea and J. H. Yardley: *American Journal of Pathology, 52:* 1191–1206, 1968.)

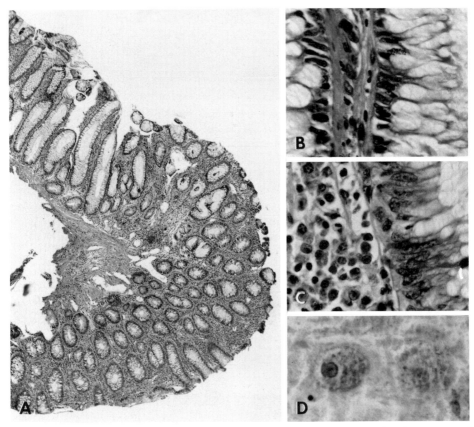

FIG. 21. Colo-rectal biopsy in a patient with chronic amebiasis. Except for the presence of organisms, the histologic findings are not distinguishable from those seen in other forms of inflammatory bowel disease. *A*, overview to show patchy, almost focal inflammation. × 35. *B*, detail from area that was only slightly inflamed. Epithelial mucin is abundant. × 450. *C*, area showing nonspecific inflammation and depletion of epithelial mucin. × 450. *D*, probable *Entamoeba histolytica* organisms in the exudate which overlay the mucosa (diagnosis confirmed by stool examination). × 900.

for diagnosing amebic dysentery since it cannot match the yield of 90% or better from the optimal use of stool smears,[3, 64] but the chance of making the diagnosis in biopsies is still good.[36, 64] Organisms are found most readily in the inflammatory exudate overlying the mucosa (Fig. 21, *D*) or in the superficial part of ulcers rather than deep within the tissue.[36, 65] Staining by PAS, Masson, and phosphotungstic acid hematoxylin methods help in recognizng the organisms and in distinguishing them from macrophages and sloughed epithelial cells. Trophozoites of *Entamoeba histolytica* cannot be distinguished with complete reliability from nonpathogenic *Entamoeba coli* in tissue sections, but organisms related to inflammation and showing compatible nuclear and cytoplasmic details (Fig. 21, *D*) permit amebiasis to be strongly suggested.

Balantidiasis is a rare acute or chronic form of colitis caused by the ciliated protozoan *Balantidium coli*.[1, 46] Most cases are found in tropical or subtropical countries among debilitated, malnourished individuals. Gross and microscopic findings in the tissue are much like those in amebiasis. The organism is readily detected in both the lumen and in the mucosa: It is so large as to dwarf the surrounding host cells.

Colitis is commonly present in chronic schistosomiasis of the Mansoni type.[46] Mucosal inflammation is caused by eggs released from adult worms that reside in the colonic vessels. The reaction to the eggs is characteristically granulomatous, but there can also be heavy infiltration by eosinophils, and much necrosis and hemorrhage is seen in the rarely noted acute phase. The granulomas (pseudotubercles) in chronic schistosomiasis form around one or more eggs and then undergo peripheral fibrosis as they heal (Fig. 22). Numerous granulomas may coalesce to give a large grossly visible submucosal nodule which sometimes ulcerates. Overgrowth of granulation tissue with the formation of pseudopolyps containing eggs also occurs. A squash preparation of the fresh biopsy tissue is a useful way to search for the eggs.

Cryptosporidiosis is caused by a coccidial organism of the genus *Cryptosporidium*. Cryptosporidia are common parasites in a variety of reptiles, birds, and mammals, but were not believed until recently to infect or to cause disease in human beings.[51, 59] A severe, acute colitis with intense acute and chronic inflam-

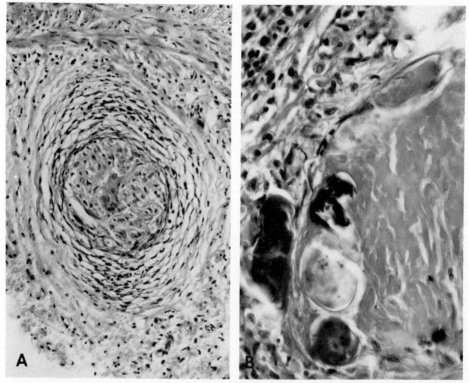

Fig. 22. Schistosomiasis. *A*, submucosal granuloma. The central mass of epithelioid cells is surrounded by a lamellated fibrous cuff containing eosinophils. × 190. *B*, a more active lesion containing eggs, some of which have calcified. × 350.

mation-surface exudation and ulceration has been seen.[59] Protozoa of the genus *Cryptosporidium* follow a life cycle comparable to other coccidia. They differ, however, from the more familiar *Isospora*, which develop within epithelial cells, in that they lie in the crypt lumens attached to the epithelial surface (Fig. 23). Because *Cryptosporidia* cannot be recognized in stool specimens, a biopsy or mucosal scraping is needed to make the diagnosis. One possible reason that cryptosporidiosis in human beings was undetected for so long is that these procedures are not performed routinely in acute enteritis and colitis.

Viral IBD. IBD due to *lymphopathia venereum* (actually a chlamydial organism) is principally a disease of females.[9] The infection begins in the genital tract and is thought to spread to the rectum via the lymphatic vessels. The deeper tissues are most heavily involved and rectal stricture may be the most prominent clinical finding. While nonspecific inflammation is usually pronounced, granulomas are a characteristic histologic finding and may show central necrosis when the disease is active.[72] There may also be ulceration and inflammation at later stages. Squamous metaplasia of the colonic mucosa occurs in *lymphopathia venereum* and when found suggests the diagnosis.

Cytomegalovirus (CMV) colitis has been described as both a primary entity[69, 79] and as a complication of ulcerative colitis.[38, 88] We have also seen CMV in a biopsy from an area of ischemic colitis, and it is evident that inflamed areas and granulation tissue are a favored site for the infection. Reduced host resistance brought on by general debility and diminished effectiveness of the immune system caused by either immunosuppressive drugs or a disease process are important factors favoring CMV colitis, as with CMV infection elsewhere.[38] Intense, nonspecific inflammation, sometimes with erosions and ulcerations, and cells having huge nuclei and prominent nuclear inclusions are the characteristic findings by rectal biopsy in CMV colitis. The involved cells are most probably macrophages[38, 69] (Fig. 24), but may look like endothelial cells when seen in small vessels. The epithelium does not show inclusions.

The large bowel has not been studied in acute nonbacterial gastroenteritis (see Chapter 4). It is entirely conceivable, however, that when such studies are performed other types of viral colitis will be identified.

Fungal IBD. Histoplasmosis is the most significant fungus infection causing IBD. It is a rare entity which can be chronic and severe; multiple pseudopolyps in the small and large intestine may be a striking finding. Biopsy will show inflammation that is both nonspecific and granulomatous. Foamy macrophages with intracellular *Histoplasma capsulatum* accumulate in the lamina propria and submucosa.[40] Since the organisms are PAS positive, the macrophages may be mistaken for muciphages.

Drug, Chemical, and Foodstuff-related IBD. It has long been known that broad spectrum antibiotics can cause a severe form of colitis in which pseudomembrane formation is often prominent.[58, 68] Tetracyclines and chloramphenicol were originally implicated; ampicillin, lincomycin, and clindamycin have received attention more recently. Some cases of antibiotic colitis, especially those associated with tetracyclines, may be related to overgrowth of a resistant strain of *Staphylococcus aureus*.[12, 58] If due to staphylococci, the process develops during treatment, and withdrawal of the offending antibiotic leads to cessation

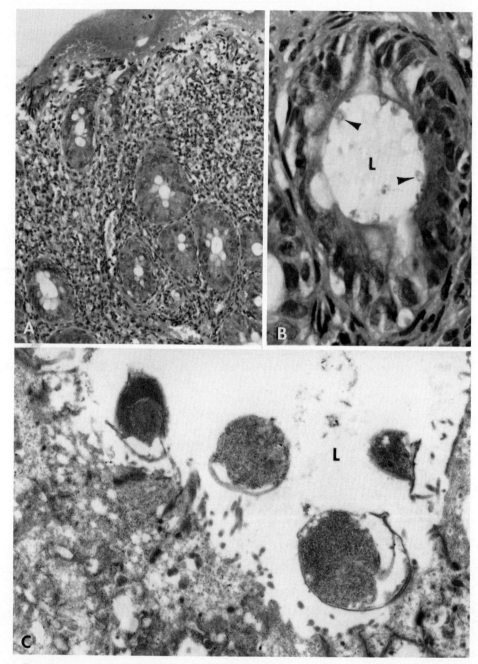

Fig. 23. Acute cryptosporidiosis. *A*, overview of inflamed mucin-depleted mucosa. × 40. *B*, a crypt showing numerous cryptosporidia in its lumen (*L*). They are mostly attached to the epithelial cells (*e. g., at arrowheads*) × 750. *C*, electron micrograph from area of crypt lumen (*L*). Multiple cryptosporidial organisms are seen. × 12,000. (Fig. A reproduced with permission from: F. A. Nime, J. D. Burek, D. L. Page, M. A. Holscher, and J. H. Yardley: *Gastroenterology 70*: 592–598, 1976.)

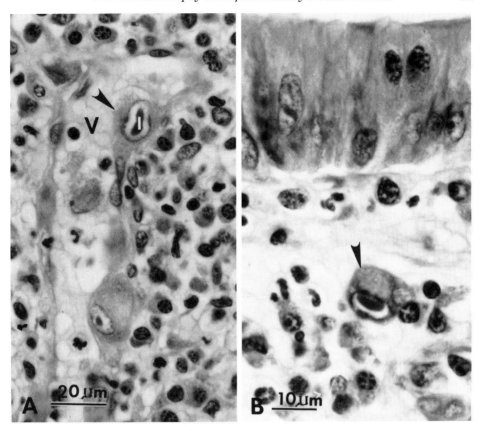

FIG. 24. Rectal biopsy showing changes of cytomegalovirus colitis. *A*, a large cell (*arrow*) with a prominent intranuclear inclusion (*I*) is found on the luminal surface of a small vessel (*V*). By electron microscopy the infected cells appeared to be macrophages rather than endothelial cells. There is also acute and chronic inflammation. × 750. *B*, a large cell (*arrowhead*), presumably a macrophage, lies in the lamina propria. It, too, demonstrates a characteristic intranuclear inclusion of cytomegalovirus infection. The overlying epithelium is mucin depleted. × 1200. (Reproduced with permission from: D. F. Keren, F. D. Milligan, J. D. Strandberg, and John H. Yardley: *The Johns Hopkins Medical Journal, 136:* 178–182, 1975.)

of symptoms. But in many patients the manner in which antibiotics causes colitis is not clear. Furthermore, clindamycin colitis can develop from a few days to several weeks after completion of treatment.[82] Altered stool bile salts,[6] ischemia (see Chapter 2), and superinfection by a virus[77] have also been suggested as pathogenetic factors, but such observations will require confirmation.

Grossly, the pseudomembrane of antibiotic colitis may be diffuse or distributed as multiple discrete plaques, the latter form being especially common following lincomycin or clindamycin (Fig. 25, *A*).[82] Histologically, mucin hypersecretion, along with inflammation and necrosis, are often prominent features of the pseudomembrane. In some cases of lincomycin and clindamycin colitis we have found evidence of mucus hypersecretion without a pseudomembrane (Fig. 25, *B*), and demonstration of a pseudomembrane grossly or in the

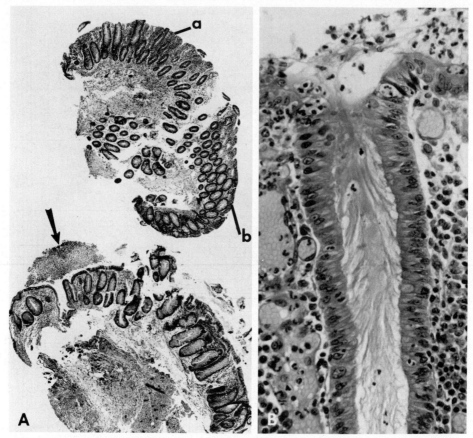

Fig. 25. Antibiotic colitis. *A*, overview of biopsy specimen from a patient who received clinda-mycin. The inflammation here is very patchy in distribution (compare area *a* and *b*). Pseudomem-brane formation (*arrow*) is characteristically plaque-like but is often not detected histologically. ×
25. *B*, mucus secretion may be prominent in clindamycin colitis, as in this crypt. Inflammatory exudate is present on the surface. × 320.

histologic material is not a *sine qua non*. The pseudomembrane may also be missing because of detachment from the specimen before sectioning, or because the biopsy specimen came from the mucosa between the lesions.

The intestinal epithelium is potentially susceptible to a variety of cytotoxic drugs, as would be anticipated from their rapid turnover and high metabolic and synthetic activities. When changes in the colo-rectal mucosa induced by one cytoxic drug, 5-hydroxyuracil (5-FU), were studied, there was gross reddening and friability, and histologically there was epithelial damage with nuclear hyperchromatism and associated acute and chronic inflammation.[17, 52] Frank mucosal necrosis occurred in some patients, but mucosal response to 5-FU varied and correlation between symptoms and histologic changes was not close.[52]

Both inorganic mercury and arsenic compounds cause an acute IBD.[44] Mer-cury poisoning was commonly seen when Calomel (HgCl) was a widely used drug and when the far more toxic mercuric chloride ($HgCl_2$) was available as a household and industrial compound. Acute mercury poisoning presents as a nonspecific acute colitis with pseudomembrane formation.[44] Chronic inorganic mercury poisoning can also develop after prolonged use of Calomel as a laxative, and is typically superimposed on severe melanosis coli. For reasons that are not clear, but which could conceivably relate to ischemia, the patient may develop an acute colitis (Fig. 26). The inorganic mercury is heavily deposited in the tissues as black mercuric sulfide crystals that are specifically associated with the pseudomelanin granules (Fig. 27).[85] The possibility should be explored that this entity is related to cathartic colon[56] since that condition has also shown a combination of heavy laxative use, melanosis coli, colitis, and possibly neurologic changes.

Cow's milk is the foodstuff that has received most attention as a possible cause of proctocolitis. Soy milk may also lead to proctitis,[29] and other foods will undoubtedly be implicated in time. Clinical and histologic changes that are indistinguishable from ulcerative colitis have been attributed to milk protein in infants, presumably on an allergic basis.[30] Milk can also adversely affect patients with idiopathic ulcerative colitis, but allergy is not the mechanism by which this usually occurs. Instead, hyperosmolar effects and lactic acid produced by bacteria in patients with coincidental lactase deficiency lead to intensification of preexisting colitis.[78]

Irradiation Colitis. IBD can develop as an acute reaction to ionizing irradia-

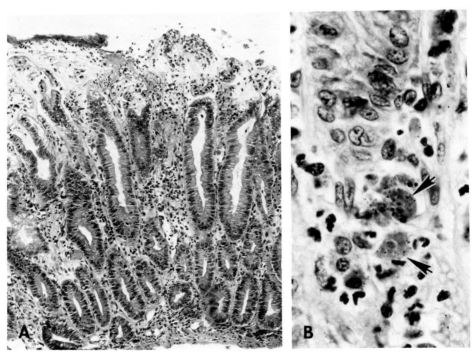

FIG. 26. Acute colitis in a patient with chronic inorganic mercury poisoning due to long-standing use of Calomel. *A*, there is marked acute inflammation with surface exudate, mucin depletion, and crypt damage. × 45. *B*, pigmented macrophages of melanosis coli (*arrows*) are present along with the acute inflammation. × 750.

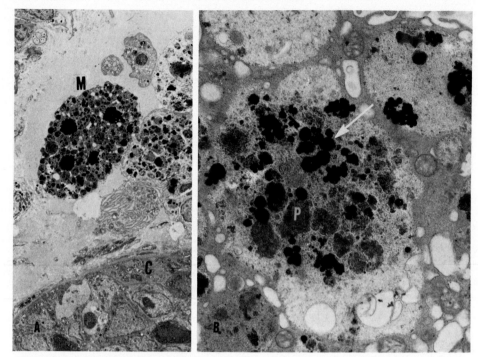

FIG. 27. Electron microscopic findings in chronic inorganic mercury poisoning. *A*, a macrophage containing pseudomelanin (*M*) is seen in the lamina propria near a crypt (*C*). × 1650. *B*, detail of pseudomelanin granules. They contain typical granular and membranous material of varying density as at *P*. The ultrastructure is unusual, however, in that ultradense deposits (*arrow*) are associated with the membranous aggregates. The ultradense deposits were demonstrated by electron diffraction to correspond to black (beta) mercuric sulfide. × 14,250. (Reproduced with permission from: J. R. Wands, S. W. Weiss, J. H. Yardley, and W. C. Maddrey: *The American Journal of Medicine 57*: 92–101, 1974.)

tion during or immediately after exposure; the small intestine is probably more sensitive than the colon and rectum. Gelfand *et al.*[23] studied rectal biopsies in 11 patients who were receiving up to 5600 rad to the pelvic area. Endoscopic alterations developed in about half, and most patients showed histologic damage to surface and crypt epithelium. There was reduced mucin, and mitotic figures were decreased in number. An unusual, regularly noted feature was crypt abscesses that were composed almost entirely of eosinophils.[23, 87] Epithelial atypia may be marked[87] (Fig. 28). Acute changes disappear and the rectal mucosa returns towards normal in most patients by 1 month after completion of therapy. In the study of Gelfand *et al.*[23] one of 11 patients later showed mucosal atrophy and there was increased epithelial mucin in others.

Postirradiation IBD can appear any time from a few weeks to many years after exposure.[7, 62] The resulting lesion can vary widely in severity. In severe cases ulceration, thickening of the wall, and associated stricture formation develop.[7] Study of autopsy and surgical resection material has shown characteristic changes in the connective tissue, including hyaline thickening of the collagen and abnormal fibroblasts. Telangiectasias are also observed along with various forms of vascular sclerosis, and subendothelial foam cells may be found in larger vessels.[62,76,86] DeCosse *et al.*[13] noted more frequent occurrence of hypertension, diabetes mellitus, and arteriosclerosis in patients with postirradiation IBD. These authors theorized that the onset of cardiovascular disease later in life heightened the likelihood of ischemic disease in a splanchnic circulation that was previously compromised by the irradiation effects. Thus postirradiation IBD may be a special form of ischemic bowel disease.

Colo-rectal biopsy specimens from patients with postirradiation IBD typically show diffuse or patchy nonspecific acute and chronic inflammation and varying degrees of mucosal injury. Characteristic connective tissue changes and the underlying vascular lesions related to the irradiation therapy are usually not identified, so that it is not ordinarily possible for the pathologist to do more than indicate that the changes are consistent with postirradiation colitis.

IBD of Intrinsic Origin. Ischemic colitis is discussed in Chapter 2, and only a few points that are relevant to biopsy material will be mentioned here. The findings in colo-rectal specimens from ischemic colitis are variable, being dependent on such features as vessel size and distribution, presence of permanent vs. temporary ischemic occlusion, the period of ischemia, and the time interval between the onset of ishcemia and biopsy.[47] Gangrenous changes of recent onset will show total necrosis of the mucosa (Fig. 29). In this form the lesion is easy to recognize as having an ischemic origin although we have seen erroneous attribution of mucosal changes to autolysis when inflammation was absent. Hemorrhage is often prominent, especially in the severe gangrenous lesion. On the other hand, biopsy specimens from milder or incomplete forms of ischemic colitis

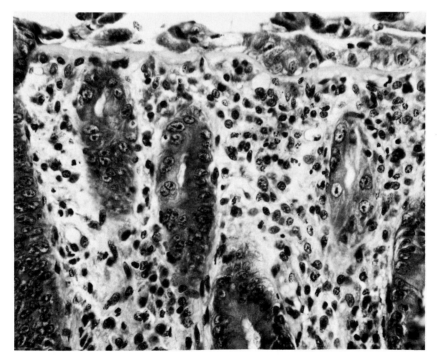

FIG. 28. Acute irradiation proctitis in a woman undergoing treatment of cervical carcinoma. In addition to acute and chronic inflammation, there is marked atypia of crypt epithelium. × 325.

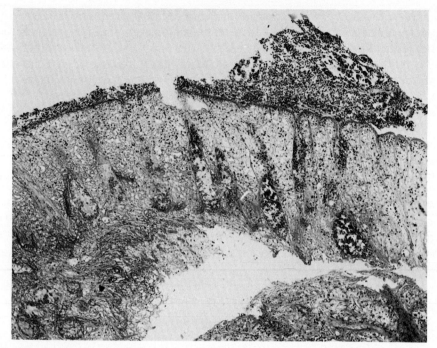

FIG. 29. Advanced necrosis in ischemic colitis. The mucosa is hemorrhagic and crypts are mostly seen in ghost outline. Surface inflammatory exudate is also present. × 35.

show findings that are nonspecific. Acute and chronic inflammation, pseudo-membrane formation, necrosis, erosion or ulceration, and epithelial regeneration can be found in various combinations. Fibrin thrombi are sometimes noted in the small submucosal and mucosal vessels. Recent studies suggest, however, that capillary thrombi are a secondary nonspecific feature.[5] Biopsy material from the mucosa overlying healed or stenotic ischemic lesions may show prominent fibrosis[67] and other changes suggesting inactive IBD.

The solitary ulcer syndrome[45, 56, 71] is a lesion which has not received the attention it surely deserves as an occasional problem in the differential diagnosis of IBD. The lesion, which is not necessarily either solitary or ulcerated, occurs on the anterior rectal wall at 7–10 cm. from the anal margin. Cardinal diagnostic features are epithelial hyperplasia, sometimes with extension of glands into the submucosa, and infiltration of the lamina propria by smooth muscle cells and fibroblasts (Fig. 30). The lesion has on occasion been mistaken for adenocarcinoma. Straining at stool, rectal prolapse, trauma, and ischemia may be causative factors.[71] The solitary ulcer syndrome may well be identical to localized colitis cystica profunda, hamartomatous inverted polyp, and the descending perineal syndrome.[56, 71]

The inflammatory changes in diverticulitis are confined to the diverticula and the pericolic tissues.[54] A mucosal biopsy typically shows, therefore, no inflammation at even a short distance from the opening of an inflamed diverticulum, and by demonstrating normal mucosa, colo-rectal biopsy in diverticulitis can be used to help rule out the presence of another disorder. On the other hand, when

Crohn's disease is present in an area where there is also diverticulosis, it may be erroneously concluded that the patient has diverticulitis.[73] In this situation mucosal biopsy from the vicinity of the diverticular disease and rectum can lead to a correct diagnosis. True diverticulitis and Crohn's disease occurring in the same individual have also been described.[22]

Patients with obstruction due to tumor[33] or other cause may develop an acute, nonspecific, ulcerating, necrotizing colitis proximal to the narrowing. Hirschsprung's disease is an important situation where this complication may be noted. The enterocolitis in Hirschsprung's disease is particularly life-threatening in the neonatal period and can present a serious diagnostic enigma.[4] Vascular insufficiency and bacterial enterocolitis with Swartzmann reaction have been suggested as possible mechanisms under these circumstances.[4]

Pseudomembranous Enterocolitis. This term is widely used to describe severe acute enteritis in which pseudomembrane formation is a prominent finding. Varied opinions have been expressed as to the cause(s) of pseudomembranous enterocolitis. These have included heavy metal poisoning, uremia, staphylococcal overgrowth, septicemia, bacillary dysentery, paratyphoid fever, shock, antibiotics, corticosteroid therapy, obstruction, postoperative states, and irradiation.[28] It is evident that most of the listed causes or associations have been discussed in the previous sections of this review. In all likelihood ischemia is a

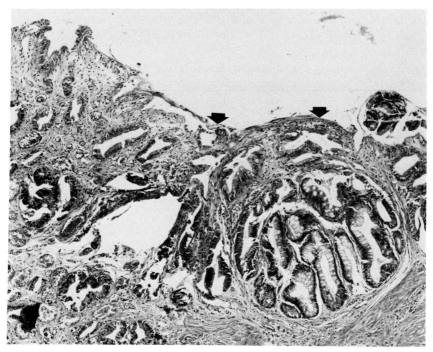

FIG. 30. Rectal lesion in the solitary ulcer syndrome. There is erosion (*arrows*) and the glands are hyperplastic and have regenerated in a very irregular fashion. Also, smooth muscle and fibrous tissue have largely replaced the lamina propria. × 170.

factor in many situations where a pseudomembranous colitis develops (see Chapter 2), particularly in systemic abnormalities such as shock, uremia, and septicemia, but there are undoubtedly other factors also. Goulston and McGovern[28] stressed the possibility that intraluminal substances might be important. From a practical standpoint, the main consideration is to avoid the notion that pseudomembranous enterocolitis is a separate, distinct entity. Instead it is a descriptive term which is applicable to many forms of IBD.

SUMMARY

The term inflammatory bowel disease (IBD) is viewed as all-inclusive, covering the full panoply of intestinal disorders in which inflammatory changes are a prominent feature, including those of infectious, toxic, and intrinsic origin, as well as the idiopathic entities ulcerative colitis and Crohn's disease.

This chapter describes and discusses those aspects of colo-rectal biopsy in IBD which can help pathologists make optimal interpretations. The areas covered are: 1) methods used to prepare biopsy specimens for study, 2) normal histologic findings and common artefacts, 3) basic pathologic changes occurring in IBD, 4) a general approach to differential diagnosis in IBD, and 5) discussion of the various individual forms of IBD. The importance of full and reliable information exchange between the endoscopist and pathologist is stressed.

Special attention is given to features in biopsy specimens which help in differentiating between ulcerative colitis and Crohn's disease. Other entities discussed are bacterial dysenteries; gonococcal proctitis; tuberculosis; Whipple's disease; amebiasis; balantidiasis; schistosomiasis; cryptosporidiosis; lymphopathia venereum; cytomegalovirus infection; histoplasmosis; antibiotic colitis; IBD due to cytotoxic drugs (5-FU), heavy metals, and foodstuffs; irradiation colitis; ischemic colitis; solitary ulcer syndrome; diverticulitis; and colitis secondary to obstruction. The term pseudomembranous enterocolitis is also considered.

ACKNOWLEDGMENTS

Many house officers, Fellows, and other physicans have contributed directly and indirectly to this chapter by participating in various projects over the years. Their help is greatly appreciated. We are grateful to Drs. Theodore Bayless, Thomas Hendrix, and Moses Paulson for the chance we have had to learn from their patients and from them. Numerous persons also provided technical skills, but the help of Mrs. Nancy Folker, Mr. Robert Gottschalk, Mrs. Dorothy Jay, and Mr. Edward Walker (deceased) was especially valuable. Photomicrographs were taken by Mr. Raymond E. Lund, RBP, FBPA.

REFERENCES

1. Ash, J. E., and Spitz, S.: Dysentery. In *Pathology of Tropical Diseases: An Atlas*, pp. 77–109. Washington, D.C., American Registry of Pathology, 1945. (Reprinted in 1968 by W. B. Saunders Co.).
2. Azzopardi, J. G., and Evans, D. J.: Muciprotein-containing histiocytes (muciphages) in the rectum. *J. Clin. Pathol. 19:* 368–374, 1966.
3. Barrett-Connor, E.: Amebiasis, today, in the United States. *Calif. Med. 114:* No. 3, 1–6, 1971.
4. Bill, A. H., and Chapman, N. D.: The enterocolitis of Hirschsprung's disease; its natural history and treatment. *Am. J. Surg. 103:* 70–74,1962.
5. Brandt, L. J., Gomery, P., Mitsuda, S., Chandler, P., and Bosley, S. J.: Disseminated intravascular coagulation in non-occlusive mesenteric ischemia; the lack of specificity of fibrin thrombi in intestinal infarction (abstract). *Gastroenterology 70:* 866, 1976.

6. Burbige, E. J., and Milligan, F. D.: Pseudomembranous colitis; association with antibiotics and therapy with cholestyramine. *J. A. M. A. 231:* 1157–1158, 1975.

7. Chau, P. M., Fletcher, G. H., Rutledge, F. N., and Dodd, G. D.: Complications in high dose whole pelvis irradiation in female pelvic cancer. *Am. J. Roentgenol. Radium Ther. Nucl Med. 87:* 22–40, 1962.

8. Cook, M. G., and Dixon, M. F.: An analysis of the reliability of detection and diagnostic value of various pathological features in Crohn's disease and ulcerative colitis. *Gut 14:* 255–262, 1973.

9. Coutts, W. E., Opazo, L., and Montenegro, M.: Digestive tract infection by the virus of lymphogranuloma inguinale. *Am. J. Dig. Dis. 7:* 287–293, 1940.

10. Curtis, K. J., and Sleisenger, M. H.: Infectious and parasitic diseases in: *Gastrointestinal Disease*, Chapter 104 edited by Sleisenger, M. H., and Fordtran, J. S., pp. 1369–1405. Philadelphia, W. B. Saunders Co., 1973.

11. Dawson, I. M. P.: The value for diagnosis and research of special investigation on rectal biopsies in Crohn's disease. *Br. J. Surg. 59:* 806–809, 1972.

12. Dearing, W. H., Baggenstoss, A. H., and Weed, L. A.: Studies on the relationship of *Staphylococcus aureus* to pseudomembranous enteritis and to postantibiotic enteritis. *Gastroenterology 38:* 441–451, 1960.

13. DeCosse, J. J., Rhodes, R. S., Wentz, W. B., Reagan, J. W., Dworken, H. J., and Holden, W. D.: The natural history and management of radiation induced injury of the gastrointestinal tract. *Ann. Surg. 170:* 369–384, 1969.

14. Dick, A. P., and Grayson, M. J.: Ulcerative colitis. A follow-up investigation with mucosal biopsy studies. *Br. Med. J. 1:* 160–165, 1961.

15. Dyer, N. H., Stansfeld, A. G., and Dawson, A. M: The value of rectal biopsy in the diagnosis of Crohn's disease. *Scand. J. Gastroenterol. 5:* 491–496, 1970.

16. Editorial. Rectal Biopsy. *Lancet 2:* 415–416, 1972.

17. Floch, M. H., and Hellman, L: The effect of five-fluorouracil on rectal mucosa. *Gastroenterology 48:* 430–437, 1965.

18. Folley, J. H.: Ulcerative proctitis. *N. Engl J. Med. 282:* 1362–1364, 1970.

19. Formal, S. B., LaBrec, E. H., and Schneider, A.: Pathogenesis of bacillary dysentery in laboratory animals. *Fed. Proc. 24:* 29–34, 1965.

20. Gear, E. V., and Dobbins, W. O.: Rectal biopsy; a review of its diagnostic usefulness. *Gastroenterology 55:* 522–544, 1968.

21. Geboes, K., and Vantrappen, G.: The value of colonoscopy in the diagnosis of Crohn's disease. *Gastrointest. Endosc. 22:* 18–23, 1975.

22. Gelb, A. M., and Finkelstein, W. E.: Differential diagnosis of diverticulitis and granulomatous colitis; exacerbation of granulomatous colitis after sigmoid resection. *Am. J. Gastroenterol. 62:* 9–15, 1974.

23. Gelfand, M. D., Tepper., M., Katz, L. A., Binder, H. J., Yesner, R., and Floch, M.: Acute irradiation proctitis in man; development of eosinophilic crypt abscesses. *Gastroenterology 54:* 401–411, 1968.

24. Gilman, R. H., and Prathap, K.: Acute intestinal ameobiasis-proctoscopic appearances with histopathological correlation. *Ann. Trop. Med. Parasitol. 65:* 359–365, 1971.

25. Gonzalez-Licea, A., and Yardley, J. H.: A comparative ultrastructural study of the mucosa in idiopathic ulcerative colitis, shigellosis and other human colonic diseases. *Bull. Johns Hopkins Hosp. 118:* 444–461, 1966.

26. Gonzalez-Licea, A., and Yardley, J. H.: Nature of the tissue reaction in ulcerative colitis; light and electron microscopic findings. *Gastroenterology 51:* 825–838, 1966.

27. Gonzalez-Licea, A., and Yardley, J. H.: Whipple's disease in the rectum; light and electron microscopic findings. *Am. J. Pathol. 52:* 1191–1206, 1968.

28. Goulston, S. J. M., and McGovern, V. J.: Pseudo-membranous colitis. *Gut 6:* 207–212, 1965.

29. Greenberger, N., and Gryboski, J. D.: Allergic disorders of the intestine and eosinophilic gastroenteritis. In *Gastrointestinal Diseases*, Chapter 81, edited by Sleisenger, M. H., and Fordtran, J. S., pp. 1066–1082. Philadelphia, W. B. Saunders Co., 1973.

30. Gryboski, J. D., Burkle, F., and Hillman, R.: Milk induced colitis in an infant. *Pediatrics 38:* 299–302, 1966.

31. Hellstrom, H. R., and Fisher, E. R.: Estimation of mucosal mucin as an aid in the differentiation of Crohn's disease of the colon and chronic ulcerative colitis. *Am. J. Clin. Pathol. 48:* 259–268, 1967.

32. Hendrix, T. R. and Yardley, J. H.: Whipple's disease. In *Modern Trends in Gastro-enterology*, Chapter 11, edited by Card, W. I., and Creamer, B., vol. 4, pp. 229–251. London, Butterworth, 1970.

33. Hurwitz, A., and Khafif, R. A.: Acute necrotizing colitis proximal to obstructing neoplasms of the colon. *Surg. Gynecol. Obstet. 111:* 749–752, 1960.

34. Johnson, W. D., and Roth, J. L. L.: Diagnosis and differential diagnosis of chronic ulcerative colitis and Crohn's colitis. In *Inflammatory Bowel Disease*, Chapter 14, edited by Kirsner, J. B., and Shorter, R. G., pp. 201–224. Philadelphia, Lea & Febiger, 1975.

35. Jones, J. H., Lennard-Jones, J. E., Morson, B. C., Chapman, M., Sackin, M. J., Sneath, P. H. A., Spicer, C. C., and Card, W. I.: Numerical taxonomy and discriminant analysis applied to nonspecific colitis. *Q. J. Med. 42:* 715–732, 1973.

36. Juniper, K., Steele, V. W., and Chester, C. L.: Rectal biopsy in the diagnosis of amebic colitis. *South Med. J. 51:* 545–553, 1958.

37. Kent, T. H., Formal, S. B., and LaBrec, E. A.: Salmonella gastroenteritis in rhesus monkeys. *Arch. Pathol. 82:* 272–279, 1966.

38. Keren, D. F., Milligan, F. D., Strandberg, J. D., and Yardley, J. H.: Intercurrent cytomegalovirus colitis in a patient with ulcerative colitis. *Johns Hopkins Med. J. 136:* 178–182, 1975.

39. Kilpatrick, Z. M.: Gonorrheal proctitis. *N. Engl. J. Med. 287:* 967–969, 1972.

40. Kirk, M. E., Lough, H. J., and Warner, H. A.: Histoplasma colitis; an electron microscopic study. *Gastroenterology 61:* 46–54, 1971.

41. Kirsner, J. B., and Shorter, R. G: *Inflammatory bowel disease*. Philadelphia, Lea & Febiger, 1975.

42. Lumb, G., and Protheroe, R. H. B.: Ulcerative colitis; a pathologic study of 152 surgical specimens. *Gastroenterology 34:* 381–407, 1958.

43. Lutzker, L. G., and Factor, S. M.: Effects of some water-soluble contrast media on the colonic mucosa. *Radiology 118:* 545–548, 1976.

44. MacCallum, W. G.: *A Textbook of Pathology*. 7th ed., pp. 389–392. Philadelphia, W. B. Saunders Co., 1941.

45. Madigan, M. R. and Morson, B. C.: Solitary ulcer of the rectum. *Gut 10:* 871–881, 1969.

46. Marcial-Rojas, R. A. (editor): *Pathology of protozoal and helminthic diseases*. Baltimore, Williams & Wilkins, 1971.

47. Marston, A., Pheils, M. T., Thomas, M. L., and Morson, B. C.: Ischaemic colitis, *Gut 7:* 1–15, 1966.

48. Matts, S. G. F.: The value of rectal biopsy in the diagnosis of ulcerative colitis. *Q. J. Med. 30:* 393–407, 1961.

49. McGovern, V. J.: The differential diagnosis of colitis. In *Pathology Annual, 1969*, edited by Sommers, S. C., vol. 4, pp. 127–158. New York, Appleton-Century-Crofts, 1969.

50. Meisel, J. L., Bergman, D., Saunders, D. R., and Graney, D.: Human rectal mucosa; proctoscopic and morphologic changes caused by laxatives (abstract). *Gastroenterology 70:* 918, 1976.

51. Meisel, J. L. Perera, D. R., Meligro, C., and Rubin, C. E.: Overwhelming watery diarrhea associated with a cryptosporidium in an immunosuppressed patient. *Gastroenterology 70:* 1156–1160, 1976.

52. Milles, S. S., Muggia, A. L., and Spiro, H. M.: Colonic histologic changes induced by 5-fluorouracil. *Gastroenterology 43:* 391–399, 1962.

53. Moore, K. L., Graham, M. A., and Barr, M. L.: The detection of chromosomal sex in hermaphrodites from a skin biopsy. *Surg. Gynecol. Obstet. 96:* 641–648, 1953.

54. Morson, B. C.: Pathology of diverticular disease of the colon. *Clin. Gastroenterol. 4:* 37–52, 1975.

55. Morson, B. C.: Rectal biopsy in inflammatory bowel disease. *N. Engl. J. Med. 287:* 1337–1339, 1972.

56. Morson, B. C.: The technique and interpretation of rectal biopsies in inflammatory bowel disease. In *Pathology Annual*, edited by Sommers, S. C., pp. 209–230. New York, Appleton-Century-Crofts, 1974.

57. Mottet, N. K.: *Histopathologic spectrum of regional enteritis and ulcerative colitis*. Philadelphia, W. B. Saunders Co. 1971.

58. Newman, C. R.: Pseudomembranous enterocolitis and antibiotics. *Ann. Intern. Med. 45:* 409–444, 1956.

59. Nime, F. A., Burek, J. D., Page, D. L., Holscher, M. A., and Yardley, J. H.: Acute enterocolitis in a human being infected with the protozoan cryptosporidium. *Gastroenterology 70:* 592–598, 1976.

60. Paustian, F. F., and Monto, G. L.: Tuberculosis of the intestine. In *Gastroenterology*, Chapter 76, edited by Bockus, H. L., 3rd ed., vol. 2, pp. 750–777. Philadelphia, W. B. Saunders Co., 1976.

61. Pearse, A. G. E: *Histochemistry: Theoretical and Applied*, 2nd ed., p. 338. Boston, Little, Brown & Co., 1960.

62. Pessel, J. F.: Irradiation bowel injury (rectal ulcer, factitial proctitis, sigmoiditis, and enteritis). In *Gastroenterology*, edited by Bockus, H. L., 2nd ed., vol. II, pp. 1042–1050. Philadelphia, W. B. Saunders Co., 1964.

63. Pike, B. F., Phillippi, P. J., and Lawson, E. H.: Soap colitis. *N. Engl. J. Med. 285:* 217–218, 1971.

64. Pittman, F. E., El-Hashimi, W. K., and Pittman, J. C.: Studies of human amebiasis. I. Clinical and laboratory findings in eight cases of acute amebic colitis. *Gastroenterology 65:* 581–587, 1973.

65. Pittman, F. E., El-Hashimi, W. K., and Pittman J. C.: Studies of human amebiasis. II. Light and electron microscopic observation of colonic mucosa and exudate in acute amebic colitis. *Gastroenterology 65:* 588–603, 1973.

66. Prathap, K., and Gilman, R.: The histopathology of acute intestinal amebiasis; a rectal biopsy study. *Am. J. Pathol. 60:* 229–246, 1970.

67. Price, A. B., and Morson, B. C.: Inflammatory bowel disease; the surgical pathology of Crohn's disease and ulcerative colitis. *Hum. Pathol. 6:* 7–29, 1975.

68. Reiner, L., Schlesinger, M. J., and Miller, G. M.: Pseudomembranous colitis following aureomycin and chloramphenicol. *Arch. Pathol. 54:* 39–67, 1952.

69. Rosen, P., Armstrong, D., and Price, N.: Gastrointestinal cytomegalovirus infection. *Arch. Intern. Med. 132:* 274–276, 1973.

70. Rout, W. R., Formal, S. B., Giannella, R. A., and Dammin, G. J.: Pathophysiology of shigella diarrhea in the rhesus monkey; intestinal transport, morphological, and bacteriological studies. *Gastroenterology 68:* 270–278, 1975.

71. Rutter, K. R. P., and Riddel, R. H.: The solitary ulcer syndrome of the rectum. *Clin. Gastroenterol. 4:* 505–530, 1975.

72. Saad, E. A., deGouveia, O. F., Filho, P. D., Teixeira, D., Pereira, A. A., and Erthal, A.: Ano-recto-colonic lymphogranuloma venereum. *Gastroenterologia 97:* 89–102, 1962.

73. Schmidt, G. T., Lennard-Jones, J. E., Morson, B. C., and Young, A. C.: Crohn's disease of the colon and its distinction from diverticulitis. *Gut 9:* 7–16, 1968.

74. Schmitt, M. G., Wu, W. C., Geenen, J. E., and Hogan, W. J.: Diagnostic colonoscopy; an assessment of the clinical indications. *Gastroenterology 69:* 765–769, 1975.

75. Sessions, J. T.: *Inflammatory bowel disease; viewpoints on digestive disease*, vol 7, no. 4. Durham, N.C., American Gastroenterological Association, September 1975.

76. Sheehan, J. F.: Foam cell plaques in the intima of irradiated small arteries (one-hundred to five-hundred microns in external diameter). *Arch. Pathol. 37:* 297–308, 1944.

77. Steer, H. W.: The pseudomembranous colitis associated with clindamycin therapy — a viral colitis. *Gut 16:* 695–706, 1975.

78. Struthers, J. E., Singleton, J. W., and Kern, F.: Intestinal lactase deficiency in ulcerative colitis and regional ileitis. *Ann. Intern. Med. 63:* 221–228, 1965.

79. Tamura, H.: Acute ulcerative colitis associated with cytomegalic inclusion virus. *Arch. Pathol. 96:* 164–167, 1973.

80. Tawile, N. T., Priest, R. J., and Schuman, B. M.: Colonoscopy in inflammatory bowel disease. *Gastrointest. Endosc. 22:* 177–184, 1975.

81. Teague, R. H., and Read, A. E.: Polyposis in ulcerative colitis. *Gut 16:* 792–795, 1975.

82. Tedesco, F. J., Barton, R. W., and Alpers, D. H.: Clindamycin-associated colitis; a prospective study. *Ann. Intern. Med. 81:* 429–433, 1974.

83. Truelove, S. C. and Richards, W. C. D.: Biopsy studies in ulcerative colitis. *Br. Med. J. 1:* 1315–1318, 1956.
84. Volpicelli, N. A., Salyer, W. R., Milligan, F. D., Bayless, T. M., and Yardley, J. H.: The endoscopic appearance of the duodenum in Whipple's disease. *Johns Hopkins Med J. 138:* 19–23, 1976.
85. Wands, J. R., Weiss, S. W., Yardley, J. H., and Maddrey, W. C.: Chronic inorganic mercury poisoning due to laxative abuse; a clinical and ultrastructural study. *Am. J. Med. 57:* 92–101, 1974.
86. Warren, S., and Friedman, N. B.: Pathology and pathologic diagnosis of radiation lesions in the gastro-intestinal tract. *Am. J. Pathol. 18:* 499–514, 1942.
87. Weisbrot, I. M., Liber, A. F., and Gordon, B. S.: The effects of therapeutic radiation on colonic mucosa. *Cancer 36:* 931–940, 1975.
88. Wong, T-W., and Warner, N. E.: Cytomegalic inclusion disease in adults; report of 14 cases with review of literature. *Arch. Pathol. 74:* 403–422, 1962.

Chapter 6

The Precursor Tissue of Ordinary Large Bowel Cancer: Implications for Cancer Prevention*

NATHAN LANE

Trying to trace the origin of large bowel neoplasia by morphologic means has been a main interest in our laboratory for many years. The only benign lesions needing consideration are hyperplastic polyps and adenomas. Furthermore, since the great majority of large bowel cancers are moderate and well differentiated adenocarcinomas, our concern is only with these. The rare, undifferentiated carcinomas following ulcerative colitis are not considered. Some insights gained from the study of familial polyposis are highly relevant to the problem.

BASIC ANATOMIC DEFINITIONS

The evolution of large bowel carcinoma via its precursor tissue is best understood by recalling some normal features. The colonic mucosa is flat and has simple test-tube glands, the crypts of Lieberkühn. The muscularis is a crucial boundary line. A neoplasm above the m. mucosae is intramucosal. A neoplasm that genuinely breaks through the m. mucosae is invasive, and may metastasize.[4] It is very important to remember the m. mucosae.

Cell division is very active, but normally is restricted to the deep one-third of the crypts (Fig. 1, A). The epithelial cells undergo upward migration and differentiate into two main cell types: the goblet cells and the absorptive cells. As shown many times with thymidine, this cell division is perfectly balanced in a number of days by exfoliation from the free surface.

If, in one or several crypts, this balance between cell division and exfoliation is somehow altered so as to favor the focal accumulation of epithelial cells, a protrusion or polyp will result.

Minute protrusions in the 1 to 3 mm. range are the commonest of all. They may be single or multiple. From various studies it seems that they may be found in 25 to 50% of asymptomatic older adults who are examined on a regular basis.[3, 6] While it is conceivable that one of these could be a tiny adenoma, one can be about 95% certain that these minute lesions, when they occur sporadically, are hyperplastic polyps.

* Reproduced from N. Lane: The Precursor Tissue of Ordinary Large Bowel Cancer. *Cancer Research (Part 2) 36:* 2669, 1975, by permission of Cancer Research.

Gastrointestinal Tract

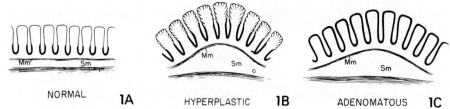

FIG. 1. *A, B, C:* The heavy shading indicates that in hyperplastic polyps, as in the normal mucosa, cell division is restricted to the deep portion of the crypts. In contrast, in adenomas, cell division is unrestricted so that mitotic figures may be observed at all levels of adenomatous tissue. Mm = muscularis mucosae; Sm = submucosa. (Reprinted with permission from: N. Lane: *Cancer Res. (Part 2) 36:* 2669, 1976.)

On the other hand, adenomas have several typical gross forms. The commonest by far is the pedunculated adenoma. It is only the head, of course, which is the neoplasm. These lesions are predominantly tubular microscopically.

Sessile adenomas are likely to be larger lesions. Sessile lesions are less common and the larger ones are typically papillary or villous microscopically. Flat or plaque-like adenomas also may be encountered. These, of course, are prototypes, and various intermediate forms can occur.

Adenomas may have a mixed tubular and villous pattern.[7] In any case, the adenomatous epithelial cells seem to be much the same in all of them.

TWO MAIN TYPES OF PROLIFERATION

In 1958[10] the difference between hyperplastic mucosal polyps and adenomas was described, and it was felt that they were readily recognizable as two distinct microscopic types. It is thought that they are biologically unrelated — that is to say, the hyperplastic polyp is not ordinarily the precursor of adenomas, and is of no consequence in the evolution of large bowel neoplasms. Hyperplastic polyps have a typical pattern of papillary hyperplasia of the epithelium, with sawtoothed glands (Figs. 2*A* and *C*). There is essentially normal differentiation into both goblet and absorptive cells.[8, 9] More important than this pattern is the fact that in hyperplastic polyps the normal repression of DNA synthesis remains intact. In other words, as shown in heavy shading in Figure 1*B*, replication remains pretty much restricted to the normal germinative zone. This emphasizes the non-neoplastic nature of these little protrusions.

On the other hand, adenomas generally do not differentiate normally into two mature cell types.[8, 9] The epithelium has a characteristic crowded picket fence appearance, and shows the usual cytologic features of neoplastic cells.[9] At the peripheral advancing edge of an adenoma, it is interesting to see how the adenomatous epithelium displaces the normal cells — always at an angle — much like a snow plow. (Figs. 2*B* and *D*). More importantly, adenomas show mitotic figures at all levels, even on the free surface, and there is extensive thymidine uptake throughout the adenomatous tissue. (Fig. 1*C*). In other words, adenomas show unrestricted replication, a feature of neoplasia, whereas in hyperplastic polyps and normal mucosa, replication is restricted.

RELATION TO CARCINOMA

Knowing the accurate classification and relative frequency of these benign lesions is essential to understand the adenoma-carcinoma sequence. The reason for this is that the frequency of all of these benign lesions is so great that no relationship of adenomatous tissue to carcinoma can be recognized without subclassifying all of them as to type, size, and relative frequency.

Accurate classification means dividing them into the non-neoplastic hyperplastic polyps and the truly neoplastic adenomas. This is usually simple for the pathologist to decide microscopically. Their relative frequency and size are shown in Table 1. This table indicates the relative frequency of these proliferations as they occur in nature, and not as a clinician would encounter them in symptomatic patients. Of 1000 proliferations, the vast majority—900 or more—

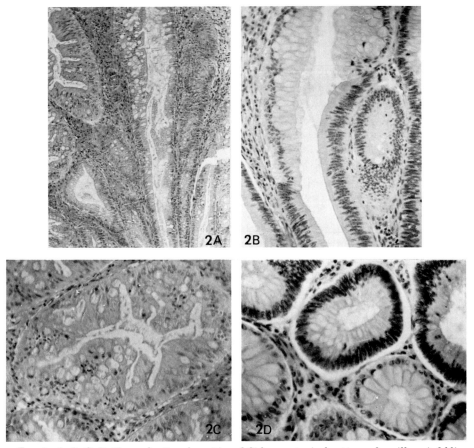

FIG. 2. *A, B, C, D:* Hyperplastic polyps (*A* and *C*) have a typical pattern of papillary infolding of the epithelium, in which both goblet and absorptive cells may be seen. Adenomatous epithelium (*B* and *D*) has a characteristic crowded picket fence appearance with marked nuclear enlargement. It fails to differentiate normally into two cell types. The contrast with normal epithelium is quite evident. (*A,* × 150; *B,* × 200; *C* and *D,* × 400). (Reprinted with permission from: N. Lane: *Cancer Res (Part 2) 36:* 2669, 1976.)

TABLE 1. CLASSIFICATION AND APPROXIMATE FREQUENCY OF RANDOMLY CHOSEN "POLYPS:"
SIGNIFICANCE OF SIZE

Of 1000 "polyps," there will be
900 hyperplastic polyps;
90 small adenomas (focal carcinoma is rare);
10 large adenomas, of which
1 will have invasive carcinoma.
Thus, incidence of invasive carcinoma = .1% in all "polyps"
but = 10% in the large adenomas

will be hyperplastic polyps.[1] There will be about 100 adenomas, but there will be only about 10 large adenomas—or about 1% of the whole group. In turn, perhaps 1 of these 10 large adenomas will have cancer in it. Thus, the chance of cancer being found in the entire group, without regard for type or size, is inconsequential, perhaps one in a thousand, or a tenth of 1%.

However, focally invasive cancer, in the subgroup of "large adenomas," occurs with sufficient frequency—about 10%—so that the large adenomas are statistically precancerous lesions. These larger adenomas with carcinoma tend to be sessile and tend to be villous, rather than tubular, microscopically. It should be remembered, however, that cancer can occur in small adenomas, but this is rare.

To arrive at the incidence with which cancer may be found in adenomas, one must remember the difference between *in situ* and invasive carcinoma. Hence, the importance of the m. mucosae in both pedunculated and sessile adenomas. Since intramucosal or *in situ* carcinoma does not metastasize, it is not clinically significant at the time of its discovery. Therefore, to be conservative, only adenomas showing invasive cancer should be counted in estimating the incidence of carcinoma in them. This distinction is also very important from the point of view of treatment of these lesions. As a rule, adenomas should be sectioned in their entirety. If one has good sections, perpendicular to the bowel wall, one can generally trace the m. mucosae, even if it follows a complex pathway.

THE QUESTION OF *"DE NOVO"* CARCINOMA

There remains some controversy as to whether carcinoma ordinarily evolves from adenomatous tissue or whether carcinoma arises *"de novo"*. A modern definition of what is meant by *"de novo* carcinoma" may be of some help. In terms of modern cell biology, the expression de novo carcinoma means that there occurs a direct one-step transformation of normal epithelial cells into microscopically recognizable cancerous epithelium and glands.

In this regard, one must keep in mind the microscopic dimensions that are involved in the cellular transformation to cancer. Therefore, only lesions measuring a few millimeters—or even less—can be accepted as possibly representing the morphology of a neoplasm at the time of its cellular origin. Thus, a 1- or 2-cm. cancer, which happens to show no residual adenomatous tissue, is not necessarily an accurate picture of the neoplasm when it was only 1 mm.—or perhaps 0.1 mm.—in size. In general, our experience has been the same as Morson's, which is that persisting adenomatous tissue is found less frequently as the size of a cancer increases.[11] In terms of cellular dimensions, by the time a cancer reaches 1 or 2 cm., it is already a large lesion. Pre-existing adenomatous tissue may well have been destroyed, and whether it is found or not in the 1 to 2 cm. size range, is pretty much irrelevant.

Carcinomas of 1 or 2 mm., or microcarcinomas, can be observed in adenomas, particularly the larger ones. However, such minute or microscopic foci of cancer, unassociated with adenomatous tissue, must be very rare, if indeed they occur at all. In spite of almost unlimited opportunity to find them, there do not seem to be any "de novo carcinomas" — in this required minute size range.

Histologic studies of familial polyposis provide valuable insight. No doubt a great deal of information is being gained by the study of animal models through the administration of a variety of carcinogens. However, familial polyposis remains mother nature's gift to the investigator. It is the natural human model for this problem since, as yet, there is no known difference in the morphogenesis of neoplasms in familial polyposis and in ordinary people.

Histologic studies in polyposis show that minute or microscopic carcinomatous foci can be found, but they occur only in adenomatous tissue. In this condition microscopic studies of many 1- to 2-mm. lesions showed only adenomas — no minute carcinomas were observed. Adenomatous changes were limited to a small number of crypts.[10]

Recently, Bussey[2] did serial sections on grossly normal areas of mucosa in specimens of polyposis. He found single crypt adenomatous change, as well as instances in which a single adjacent crypt became involved. He also found examples in which the adenomatous epithelium replaced the normal in three crypts. In cellular terms, anything as large as a tri-cryptal adenoma is already an advanced lesion — even though it is not visible grossly.

These studies seem to reveal the morphology of neoplasia at its microscopic beginning and no carcinomatous glands were seen. In brief, *de novo* carcinoma defined in modern terms of cellular dimensions has not been observed in familial polyposis, in spite of the tremendous tendency for carcinoma to develop in this condition.

It is important to be aware of the 25-year study done at the University of Minnesota Cancer Detection Center.[5] Annual sigmoidoscopic examination of a group of thousands of persons was done over many years and mucosal protrusions were removed. In over 25 years, only 11 carcinomas were found, and of these, 8 cases proved to be only focal carcinoma in adenomatous tissue. Even including these 8 as real cancer cases, the expected incidence of cancer was reduced by 85%. There seems to be no reason to doubt the validity of this study and it seems to provide strong documentation for the view that ordinary large bowel carcinoma most often develops in a precursor focus of adenomatous tissue, and not *de novo*.

To sum up this issue, the study from the University of Minnesota, the familial polyposis information, especially the work of Bussey, and the rarity of minute cancer, or microcancer in normal mucosa, vs. its occurrence in adenomatous tissue, all appear to be fundamental observations. They seem to be against the idea of *de novo* carcinoma.

Perhaps the ultimate ideal to be achieved would be to prevent the development of adenomatous tissue. Realistically, however, at the present time, in terms of preventive medicine, the safe detection and removal of adenomatous tissue seems to be the most assured way of decreasing the incidence of large bowel cancer.

CONCLUSIONS

Through the years, our aim has been to study minute lesions to clarify the morphogenesis of large bowel neoplasia. Four points are noteworthy: (1) Hyperplastic polyps and adenomas seem to be distinct and separate. (2) The larger adenomas are statistically precancerous. (3) Extensive histologic studies, both in polyposis and in ordinary humans, have not disclosed truly minute or microcancer in normal mucosa. In other words, no "de novo cancer" has been observed. One-step direct transformation of normal epithelium to cancer does not seem to be the usual pathway. (4) It seems that human polyposis is the best model for the study of large bowel neoplasia. Indeed, until new evidence appears which would downgrade human polyposis as a model, it should be the yardstick against which all other experimental results ought to be measured.

REFERENCES

1. Arthur, J. F.: Structure and significance of metaplastic nodules in the rectal mucosa. *J. Clin. Pathol. 21:* 735–743, 1968.
2. Bussey, H. J. R.: *Familial Polyposis Coli: Family studies, Histopathology, Differential Diagnosis and Results of Treatment.* Baltimore, The Johns Hopkins University Press, 1975.
3. Chapman, I.: Adenomatous polypi of large intestine; incidence and distribution. *Ann. Surg. 157:*223–226, 1963.
4. Fenoglio, C. M., Kaye, G. I., and Lane, N.: Distribution of human colonic lymphatics in normal, hyperplastic, and adenomatous tissue; its relationship to metastasis from small carcinomas in pedunculated adenomas, with two case reports. *Gastroenterology 64:* 51–66, 1973.
5. Gilbertsen, V. A.: Proctosigmoidoscopy and polypectomy in reducing the incidence of rectal cancer. *Cancer 34:* 936–939, 1974.
6. Gilbertsen, V. A., Knatterud, G. L., Lober, P. H., *et al.:* Invasive carcinoma of the large intestine: a preventable disease? *Surgery 57:* 363–365, 1965.
7. Grinnell, R. S., and Lane, N.: Benign and malignant adenomatous polyps and papillary adenomas of the colon and rectum; an analysis of 1856 tumors in 1335 patients. *Int. Abstr. Surg. 106:* 519–538, 1958.
8. Kaye, G. I., Fenoglio, C. M., Pascal. R. R., and Lane, N.: Comparative electron microscopic features of normal, hyperplastic, and adenomatous human colonic epithelium; variations in cellular structure relative to the process of epithelial differentiation. *Gastroenterology 64:* 926–945, 1973.
9. Lane, N., Kaplan, H., and Pascal, P. R.: Minute adenomatous and hyperplastic polyps of the colon; divergent patterns of epithelial growth with specific associated mesenchymal changes; contrasting roles in the pathogenesis of carcinoma. *Gastroenterology 60:* 537–551, 1971.
10. Lane, N., and Lev, R.: Observations on the origin of adenomatous epithelium of the colon; serial section studies of minute polyps in familial polyposis. *Cancer 16:* 751–764, 1963.
11. Morson, B. C.: Factors influencing the prognosis of early cancer of the rectum. *Proc. R. Soc. Med. 59:* 607–608, 1966.

Chapter 7

Polyps and Cancer of the Large Bowel

B. C. MORSON

It is well recognized that the identification of precancerous conditions is the basis of cancer prevention. At the present time isolated adenomas, familial polyposis, and ulcerative colitis are the conditions which are known to predispose to cancer of the large bowel. The concept that most cancers of the colon and rectum evolve from isolated adenomas is sometimes known as the polyp-cancer or, more accurately, the adenoma-carcinoma sequence.

Granted that a substantial body of evidence in support of the adenoma-carcinoma sequence is already available,[11] the following questions require answers: (1) Do all adenomatous polyps and villous adenomas inevitably become cancerous? (2) Do all cancers of the colon and rectum evolve from preexisting adenomatous polyps and villous adenomas? (3) How long does it take for the adenoma-carcinoma sequence to evolve? (4) If some cancers do not arise from preexisting adenomas what is the alternative mechanism of histogenesis?

THE MORPHOLOGY OF THE ADENOMA-CARCINOMA SEQUENCE

It is common to see neoplastic tumors in the colon and rectum which are partly benign and partly malignant. This can be obvious on gross examination. Sometimes, however, the benign or malignant component is only apparent as a result of microscopic studies. A macroscopically benign adenomatous polyp or villous adenoma should always be carefully examined for evidence of invasive carcinoma because the latter may be limited to small microscopic foci. Occasionally, what appears to be a benign adenomatous polyp is found to be entirely composed of carcinoma on microscopic examination (so-called polypoid carcinoma). Whatever their relative proportions the presence of contiguous benign and malignant tissue is evidence that the carcinoma arose from a previously benign adenoma.

In a series of 1961 malignant tumors seen at St. Mark's Hospital from 1957 to 1968 there were 278 (14.2%) in which there was evidence of contiguous benign tumor, either adenomatous polyp or villous adenoma. The frequency with which benign adenoma is found in continuity with a cancer varies with the extent of spread of the malignant component. If the latter has spread into the extramural tissues of the wall of the colon or rectum, the frequency with which benign tumor is found is only 7%. With spread in continuity limited to the wall of the bowel it rises to nearly 20%, but if there is invasion of the submucosal layer only it is nearly 60%. This approach to the study of the adenoma-carcinoma sequence is evidence that at least half and probably nearer two-thirds of all carcinomas of the colon and rectum arise from previously benign adenomas. It is probable that as carcinomas spread through the bowel wall they also expand on the mucosal surface and tend to destroy surviving benign tumor.

MALIGNANT POTENTIAL OF ADENOMAS

Adenomatous polyps, villous adenomas, and their synonyms are names used to describe different histologic types of benign neoplastic polyps. There is a histologic spectrum with the typical adenomatous polyp (tubular adenoma) at one end and the typical villous adenoma (villous papilloma) at the other. The intermediate histologic type has been called "papillary" adenoma and "villoglandular" or "tubulovillous" adenoma. Whatever the name used, the histologic structure is intermediate between adenomatous polyp and villous adenoma and will be described as such here.

The adenomatous polyp (75%) is far more common than the typical villous adenoma (10%) and about 15% of tumors have an intermediate structure. The malignancy rate for the different histologic types of polyp can be assessed by an analysis of the frequency with which cancer is found in a series of tumors which are either wholly or partly benign. In this context "cancer" is defined as invasion across the line of the muscularis mucosae. The general malignancy rate for the common adenomatous polyp is only 5% compared with 40% for villous adenomas. The intermediate type of polyp (often called villoglandular adenoma) with a malignant potential of 22% seems to behave more like the villous growth pattern than the adenomatous polyp. These figures emphasize that villous adenomas have much the greatest malignant potential. How can this be explained?

It has been clear for many years that there is a close relationship between size of adenomas and their malignant potential. The St. Mark's experience shows that the malignant potential of adenomatous polyps and villous adenomas (including the intermediate type) is very low indeed for tumors under 1 cm. in diameter; between 1 and 2 cm. in diameter the malignancy rate increases to 1 in 10, but nearly half of all polyps over 2 cm. in diameter contain evidence of invasive cancer. These figures obviously have great practical importance for radiologists, surgeons, and pathologists.

The common adenomatous polyp is usually small and very rarely contains invasive cancer. As they grow, however, so the malignant potential increases and about one-third of them over 2 cm. in size are malignant. But, even small villous adenomas have a malignancy rate of about 10% and cancer is found in about 50% of those over 2 cm. in diameter. The malignancy rate for the intermediate histologic type approaches much closer that for villous adenomas than that for adenomatous polyps. Mostly, the villous type of growth pattern presents as a larger tumor than the ordinary adenomatous polyp.

Although there are important differences in the frequency and behavior of adenomatous polyps, villous adenomas, and the intermediate histologic type, it must be emphasized that the cytologic characteristics in all three varieties are the same. It is essential to distinguish between the histology or tissue architecture of these tumors and their cellular features. It is customary to regard the latter as an epithelial atypia or dysplasia which can be graded as mild, moderate, or severe. Many histopathologists would regard severe dysplasia as synonymous with carcinoma-*in-situ*. However, this is an expression best avoided in the diagnostic practice of tumors of the colon and rectum because of its controversial meaning.

The grade of atypia in polyps is not always uniform and foci of severe dysplasia may be seen in a tumor which otherwise has mild or moderate dysplastic changes. The criteria for judging the degree of epithelial atypia include nuclear changes such as enlargement and pleomorphism, loss of polarity, stratification, and an increase in the number of mitotic figures, some of which may be abnormal forms. With increasing severity of dysplasia there is loss of differentiation and usually, but not invariably, a decreasing amount of mucin secretion. The diagnosis of carcinoma is made only by observing invasion across the line of the muscularis mucosae. Once this barrier has been breached there is potential for metastasis, although a distinction must be made between true carcinomatous and pseudocarcinomatous invasion.[10]

The grade of epithelial atypia is valuable in the study of the malignant potential of adenomatous polyps and villous adenomas. Mild atypia is associated with a low malignant potential, but one-third of all polyps with severe atypia contain invasive carcinoma. In other words, there is a clear correlation of increasing epithelial atypia with increasing malignant potential. The St. Mark's figures[11] also show that small adenomas very rarely show severe atypia but when they do there is a high malignant potential. But as polyps get larger the influence of the degree of atypia on malignant potential is diminished. Size seems to have paramount importance in judging the risk of cancer.

The relationship of grade of atypia to histologic type of polyp is also interesting. The malignancy rate for all adenomatous polyps with mild or moderate atypia, which are the great majority, is low. Severe atypia in adenomatous polyps is uncommon but is associated with a relatively high malignant potential (about 25%). Villous adenomas, on the other hand, often show severe atypia and this may be one important explanation for their high malignant potential compared with adenomatous polyps.

LIFE HISTORY OF THE ADENOMA-CARCINOMA SEQUENCE

The actual time it takes for the adenoma-carcinoma sequence to evolve can be measured by a study of the age distribution curves of patients with adenomas and with carcinomas. These show that adenomas appear on the average of about 4 years before carcinomas. This figure must be a considerable underestimate because, whereas the age at diagnosis of cancer may be fairly accurate, the age at diagnosis of a polyp is likely to be very approximate as they are usually symptomless. Further comment about the value of age distribution curves as applied to the adenoma-carcinoma sequence is given below under "The Adenoma-Carcinoma Sequence in Familial Polyposis."

It is rarely possible to make direct observations on the adenoma-carcinoma sequence because polyps are usually removed by local excision. The fate of 4 patients with adenomatous polyps in the rectum who refused treatment has been studied. In the first two cases the diagnosis of cancer was made about 5 years later. In the third case the adenoma-carcinoma sequence took over 12 years to evolve. The fourth patient illustrates the observation that a histologically proven adenomatous polyp may remain benign for at least 10 years without becoming malignant. It has already been shown that the malignancy rate for all adenomatous polyps is only 5%, which of course suggests that many, and probably most, adenomatous polyps never evolve into carcinoma.

It is easier to make direct observations over a long period of time on villous adenomas because these are usually large tumors which are prone to recurrence after local excision. Our studies have shown that villous tumors, proven histologically, will remain benign for up to 20 years without going malignant. In one patient benign tumor only was observed for nearly 30 years before a malignant change was detected. In another patient the evolution of the adenoma-carcinoma sequence took at least 10 years. All of these patients had repeated local excisions for benign tumor at the same site in the rectum and it is, of course, possible that this delayed the onset of carcinoma. Although it has already been shown that villous adenomas have a high malignant potential it is likely that the adenoma-carcinoma sequence, as judged by this evidence, evolves over many years and as with adenomatous polyps, it is likely that some villous adenomas may never become cancerous.

A recent study of the relationship of age of patient to epithelial atypia in adenomas and to carcinoma has shown that the average age increases with increasingly severe atypia. Moreover, the average age of patients with surgically removed carcinomas of the large bowel is greater than that for those with adenomas with the most severe grade of atypia but less than for cancers found at autopsy.[7] This confirms the progressive nature of the adenoma-carcinoma sequence. The authors also give figures which illustrate the length of time it takes for the adenoma-carcinoma sequence to evolve. This work requires confirmation but taken together with other evidence it suggests that the sequence never takes less than 5 years to evolve, usually takes 10 to 15 years, and can even cover a normal adult life span. There is probably great variability, but further support for this estimate can be obtained from a study of the adenoma-carcinoma sequence in familial polyposis.

THE ADENOMA-CARCINOMA SEQUENCE IN FAMILIAL POLYPOSIS

In this genetically predetermined condition the mucous membrane of the large intestine is covered by hundreds or thousands of adenomas. Mostly these have the structure of tubular adenomas (adenomatous polyps) but it is not sufficiently well recognized that a minority are villous and others have an intermediate histologic structure. Patients with familial polyposis will almost inevitably get cancer if left untreated and all of the evidence suggests that the carcinomas arise from the adenomas.[4]

A study of the life history of the adenoma-carcinoma sequence in familial polyposis gives very useful information which is relevant to our ideas about the time it takes for cancer to evolve from isolated adenomatous polyps or villous adenomas. For example, the age distribution curves for patients with polyposis and cancer show that the average age at diagnosis of polyposis without cancer is about 27 years and for polyposis with cancer about 39 years. This gives a time interval of about 12 years between the diagnosis of polyposis and the later development of carcinoma. As with the age distribution curves for isolated adenomas and cancers, measurement of the age at onset of polyposis is inaccurate but probably much less so than for isolated lesions. In any case the figure of 12 years is likely to be an underestimate of the length of the adenoma-carcinoma sequence in these circumstances.

More information about the time it takes for carcinoma to develop in patients with polyposis comes from analysis of the age at onset of polyposis and cancer in 59 patients who, for one reason or another, did not have any treatment for their disease. Mostly these patients were under care at St. Mark's Hospital before the operation of total colectomy and ileorectal anastomosis was established about 25 years ago. This study has shown that out of 59 patients with polyposis observed during 5 years, only 7 (12%) developed cancer. There were, then, 52 patients who harbored adenomas for 5 years without malignant change. The cancer rate between 5 and 10 years increased to 25%, but there were still 29 patients who had had adenomas for 10 years which remained benign. At 10 to 15 years the cancer rate increased to just over 30% and there were still 12 patients who had had adenomas for 15 years without any malignant change. The cancer rate at 15 to 20 years was over 50% but 4 patients had polyposis for 20 years which remained benign. Lastly, there were 3 patients in whom the adenoma-carcinoma sequence took over 20 years. These figures lend support to the concept that the evolution of carcinoma of the colon and rectum from adenomatous polyps and villous adenomas takes at least 5 years and may be more than 20 years, but on the average lies between 10 and 15 years. It must also be remembered that only one or a few cancers develop in polyposis and that most of the adenomas in this condition do not become malignant during a normal life span. It has already been shown that the malignancy rate for adenomatous polyps is only about 5%, and for villous adenomas about 40%. This must mean that many adenomatous polyps and villous adenomas never become malignant.

For many years it has been customary at St. Mark's Hospital to treat patients with familial polyposis by total colectomy and ileorectal anastomosis. The adenomas in the rectum are removed by fulguration and recurrences of benign tumor at subsequent follow-up examinations are also treated by this method. The risk of cancer in the rectal stump after colectomy and ileorectal anastomosis has been analyzed for 86 patients followed for up to 25 years. So far only 2 patients have developed cancer of the rectum at 2 and 7 years after colectomy. The longest follow-up is for 11 patients who have remained free of cancer for between 20 and 25 years. This low incidence of cancer of the rectum after colectomy and ileorectal anastomosis at St. Mark's Hospital is in great contrast to that reported from the Mayo Clinic[8] and requires some explanation. It may be significant that the rectal stump was kept free of adenomas by fulguration in all of the St. Mark's patients. In other words, removal of adenomas means prevention of cancer. It is also possible that the operation of total colectomy and ileorectal anastomosis so changes the environment of the rectal mucosa that neoplastic activity is inhibited, hence, perhaps, the observation of regression of adenomas in the rectum after this operation. The high cancer rate in the rectum in the Mayo Clinic series may, however, be explained by different methods of selection and management of patients with polyposis.

MULTIPLE BENIGN AND MALIGNANT TUMORS

There is abundant evidence that most cancers of the colon and rectum arise from previously benign adenomatous polyps and villous adenomas.[6, 9, 13, 16] Granted the importance of this relationship, a study of multiple benign and malignant tumors gives useful information about groups of patients who are at increased risk from neoplastic disease of the large bowel. Out of a total of 3002 patients at St. Mark's Hospital there were 2412 who had one tumor only and 590 (19.7%) who had multiple synchronous tumors, either benign or malignant. This means that 1 in 5 of all patients with neoplastic disease of the large bowel have more than one benign or malignant tumor somewhere in the colon or rectum. This fact has important clinical implications. It means that meticulous examination of the whole large intestine is essential for patients who have presented with a tumor in one part of it. In the same series of 3002 patients there were 210 (7%) who developed a second or metachronous benign or malignant tumor during subsequent follow-up examinations. It is probable that this figure is an underestimate because this study covers a period of time before the introduction of colonoscopy. Moreover, not all the patients had sufficiently meticulous follow-up examinations by air contrast barium enema which is essential for proper investigation of the whole colon. It is likely that the risk of a patient developing a second tumor is at least 1 in 10 and probably greater. This also illustrates the importance of follow-up of all patients who have had an adenomatous polyp, a villous adenoma, or a carcinoma removed from any part of the large intestine. Studies at St. Mark's Hospital have also shown that the risk of developing cancer increases with the number of benign adenomatous polyps or villous adenomas. At this point, the important distinction between polyps which are genuine adenomas and those which the histopathologist can recognize as hyperplastic or metaplastic polyps must be emphasized.

EPIDEMIOLOGY OF ADENOMAS

Epidemiologic studies have revealed geographic and racial differences in the incidence and mortality of cancer of the large bowel which suggest that environmental factors, such as variations in dietary habit, have etiologic importance.[2, 3, 15] In contrast, there are relatively few studies of the epidemiology and geographic pathology of adenomas of the large intestine. It is likely that environment factors affect the growth of adenomas as well as the onset and progression of invasive carcinoma. Adenomas are significantly more common in countries with a high incidence of colorectal cancer compared with low incidence areas.[1, 5, 14] Moreover, it has been shown that in high risk areas for cancer of the large bowel the adenomas are larger and show a greater propensity for the villous type of growth pattern.

In a study of the comparative histology of adenomas in England and Japan these results have been confirmed.[12] They show that the malignant potential of adenomas is the same in England and Japan when adjusted for size. In other words, individual adenomas of the same size have the same malignant potential in the two countries. The reasons why adenomas in England grow to a greater size than in Japan are unknown but it is likely that there are environmental factors involved and possibly these are the same as for invasive carcinoma.

The relative rarity of villous tumors in Japan is a striking feature of this study. Considering the fact that over 70% of adenomas examined were situated in the sigmoid colon and rectum, and the rectum is the commonest site for villous tumors, it is most unlikely that there has been any sampling error. Villous adenomas have a high malignant potential and their low prevalence in Japan is probably a main reason for the lower incidence of colorectal cancer among the Japanese. But our figures also show that tubular and tubulovillous adenomas in England have a greater malignant potential than those in Japan.

Although the three grades of epithelial atypia have the same relative incidence in the two countries, the cancer rate per grade is much greater in England than Japan. This is mostly due to the greater size of the adenomas encountered in England. The adenoma-carcinoma sequence is a progressive process through increasingly severe grades of atypia to invasive carcinoma. It would appear that the sequence operates in the same way in both countries but that the greater malignant potential of adenomas in England is mainly due to their capacity to grow to a large size. The pure villous adenoma is often a large tumor and its rarity in Japan must also be significant.

The evidence suggests that there are geographic differences in the character of adenomas which influence their potential for malignancy. Although this enquiry is based on surgical material and is not a population study, experience suggests that large bowel adenomas, like colorectal cancer, are less common in Japan than in England. However, more information is required about the geographic pathology and epidemiology of adenomas, and this could best be obtained from autopsy rather than surgical material.

CONCLUSIONS

Do all adenomatous polyps and villous adenomas inevitably became cancerous? The answer must be "*no*" if only because the prevalence of these tumors is so much greater than the prevalence of cancer. Evidence has been presented which shows that the risk of cancer varies with the size of the adenoma, with its histologic type, and with the degree of epithelial atypia. Generally speaking, the risk of cancer is very low indeed for tumors under 1 cm. in diameter but increases to 50% when the adenoma is over 2 cm. in diameter. Villous adenomas are usually larger than adenomatous polyps.

Villous adenomas have considerably greater malignant potential than adenomatous polyps. Apart from the important issue of size it has been shown that the cancer rate increases with the degree of epithelial atypia and severe atypia is more common in villous adenomas than in adenomatous polyps. However, the evidence also suggests that many adenomatous polyps and villous adenomas never become malignant.

Do all cancers of the colon and rectum evolve from preexisting adenomatous polyps and villous adenomas? The evidence suggests that the great majority of cancers of the colon and rectum have evolved through the adenoma-carcinoma sequence. If some cancers do not arise from adenomatous polyps and villous adenomas what is the alternative mechanism of histogenesis? The concept of cancer "*de novo*" is difficult to appreciate because it has never been defined in morphologic terms. It must be understood that adenomas can be very flat, although they are clearly circumscribed lesions which are only very slightly raised above the surrounding normal mucous membrane. However, it is rare for them to adopt this form in the colon and rectum. More often they are obviously elevated to form a "polyp," sessile or pedunculated.

How long does it take for the adenoma-carcinoma sequence to evolve? It is not possible to give an accurate answer, but the evidence presented here suggests that on the average it takes 10 to 15 years but it may take as little as 5 years or as long as 25 years.

There is evidence that adenomas are commoner in countries with a high incidence of colorectal cancer compared with low incidence areas. More information is required about the epidemiology of adenomas because it is likely that the evolution of the adenoma-carcinoma sequence is affected by environmental factors which operate differently in different geographic areas.

REFERENCES

1. Arminski, T. C., and McLean, D. W.: Incidence and distribution of adenomatous polyps of the colon and rectum based on 1000 autopsy examinations. *Dis. Colon Rectum.* 7: 249–261, 1964.
2. Berg, J. W., and Howell, M. A.: The geographic pathology of bowel cancer. *Cancer 34:* 807–814, 1974.
3. Burkitt, D. P., Walker, A. R. P., and Painter, N. S.: Effect of dietary fibre on stools and transit-times, and its role in the causation of disease. *Lancet 2:* 1408–1411, 1972.
4. Bussey, H. J. R.: *Familial Polyposis Coli: Family Studies, Histopathology, Differential Diagnosis and Results of Treatment.* Baltimore, The Johns Hopkins University Press, 1975.
5. Correa, P., Duque, E., Cuello, C., and Haenszel, W.: Polyps of the colon and rectum in Cali, Colombia. *Int. J. Cancer 9:* 86–96, 1972.
6. Grinnel, R. S., and Lane, N.: Benign and malignant adenomatous polyps and papillary adenomas of the colon and rectum; an analysis of 1,856 tumors in 1,335 patients. *Surg. Gynecol. Obstet 106:* 519–538, 1958.
7. Kozuka, S., Nogaki, M., Ozeki, T., and Masumori, S.: Premalignancy of the mucosal polyp in the large intestine. II. Estimation of the periods required for malignant transformation of mucosal polyps. *Dis. Colon Rectum.* 18:
8. Moertel, C. G., Hill, J. R., and Adson, M. A.: Surgical management of multiple polyposis; the problem of cancer in the retained bowel segment. *Arch. Surg. 100:* 521–526, 1970.
9. Morson, B. C., and Bussey, H. J. R.: Predisposing causes of intestinal cancer. In *Current Problems in Surgery.* Chicago, Year Book Medical Publishers, 1970.
10. Muto, T., Bussey, H. J. R., and Morson, B. C.: Pseudo-carcinomatous invasion in adenomatous polyps of the colon and rectum. *J. Clin. Pathol.* 26: 25–31, 1973.
11. Muto. T., Bussey, H. J. R. and Morson, B. C.: The evolution of cancer of the colon and rectum. *Cancer 36:* 2251–2270, 1975.
12. Muto, T.: Comparative histological study on large bowel adenomas in Japan and England with special reference to malignant potential. (To be published.)
13. Potet, F., and Soullard, J.: Polyps of the rectum and colon. *Gut 12:* 468–482, 1971.
14. Sato, E.: Adenomatous polyps of large intestine in autopsy and surgical material. *Gann 65:* 295–306, 1974.
15. Segi, M., and Kurihara, M.: *Cancer mortality for selected sites in 24 countries,* No. 6. Tokyo, Japan Cancer Society 1966–1967.
16. Welch, C. E.: Polypoid lesions of the gastrointestinal tract. Vol. II in the Series "*Major Problems in Clinical Surgery.*" Philadelphia and London, W. B. Saunders, 1964.

Chapter 8

The Precarcinomatous Lesion of Ulcerative Colitis

ROBERT H. RIDDELL

Carcinoma complicating ulcerative colitis accounts for only a very small proportion of large bowel carcinomas and the true figure is probably less than 1%. It has been estimated that there were approximately 100,000 new cases of large bowel cancers in the United States of America in 1975 (American Cancer Society, 1974), and using this figure it is estimated that only about 1000 probably arose as a complication of ulcerative colitis. It could then reasonably be asked why such a disproportionate amount of interest should be shown in these few cases. The answer is not difficult to find, for although few in number, these patients pose a real problem in management. The reasons for this are manifold but the most disturbing are that carcinomas may develop insidiously even when the patients are under active medical care, the tumors are frequently multiple, and they may not become clinically apparent until they are well advanced when only palliation can be offered. The main reason why detection can be so difficult is that many of the carcinomas complicating ulcerative colitis are flat or plaque-like (Fig. 1) and this makes them difficult to recognize either radiologically or endoscopically. This type of tumor is often very aggressive. Finally the average age at which these tumors are discovered is in the range of 40 to 45 years which is much lower than noncolitic cancers, although the average age of death (46 years) may be a more accurate index.[7] This inevitably means that many of these patients have heavy parental and financial responsibilities, while some will be in their 20's or even younger.[2] All of these factors combine to produce a problem for which there is no simple answer and this has resulted in a variety of philosophies of management. The more aggressive of these are based on the identification of a subgroup of colitics in whom virtually all of these carcinomas occur. This subgroup consists of those patients with total or extensive colitis especially with an early age of onset and a long history.

The identification of this clinical high risk group has put the clinician in a dilemma. One approach is to submit the whole of this high risk group to proctocolectomy, usually when disease has been present for 10 years. However, this wholesale sacrifice of colons has been challenged because apart from the inevitable small mortality, appreciable morbidity, and the effects of permanent ileostomy, only a small proportion of patients, even within this high risk group, would eventually develop carcinoma. It has been estimated that approximately

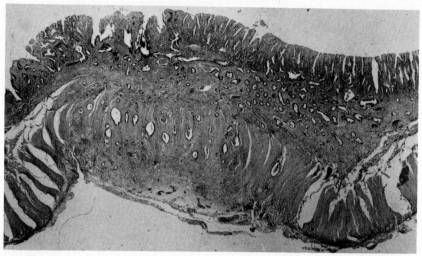

FIG. 1. Plaque-like carcinoma in ulcerative colitis. It is only slightly raised above the adjacent mucosa, but the tumor has infiltrated almost through the muscularis propria. Hematoxylin and eosin; × 14.

3.0 to 3.5% of all colitics develop cancer.[7] Since the disease in about one-fifth of all colitics is total, it follows that in this high risk group about 16% will develop carcinoma. This is in accordance with the 12.5% incidence of carcinoma at 20 years of disease indicated by Edwards and Truelove,[3] although the incidence will probably rise with the length of history. However, this incidence is considered sufficient by some to justify their aggressive management. Others see carcinoma complicating colitis so infrequently that they tend to take no special precautions. Many clinicians tend to follow a middle course and while not advocating proctocolectomy on all their high risk patients, nevertheless, become increasingly ready to advise this operation when severe exacerbations of the disease occur which they might otherwise have treated more aggressively by medical methods.

This is clearly unsatisfactory and an additional approach is required which will select those patients within this high risk clinical group who are at greatest risk from developing carcinoma, with the objective of carrying out proctocolectomy on them, or conversely, identifying those patients who seem at least risk from developing cancer so that they can merely be closely followed clinically. One such approach is to assume that these tumors go through stages of intramucosal dysplasia before becoming invasive, and to try to detect this phase by biopsy.[4, 6, 8, 9] Patients showing evidence of unequivocal dysplasia would be those who should be seriously considered for proctocolectomy, while those consistently showing no dysplasia could be followed clinically. A cancer-free population of colitics should be the objective.

TERMINOLOGY

Many of the terms used are open to subjective interpretation. The following terms define their meaning in the present context.

Precarcinomatous change — A change in the large bowel mucosa to a type which is not in itself malignant but is one from which a carcinoma will more readily arise. Scientifically, this is the most accurate term.

Premalignant change — In practice used synonymously with precarcinomatous change, but theoretically, could be used to incorporate other types of cancer arising in ulcerative colitis, *e.g.*, malignant lymphoma.

Precancerous change (precancer) — The most commonly used term. It is used synonymously with the preceding two terms but is less satisfactory because of the emotional overlay of the word cancer, which tends to be used in lay terms for any malignant process.

Atypia — Literally anything that is not typical. In this present context, any deviation from the usual acute, regenerative, or quiescent phases of ulcerative colitis. It is the broadest, and therefore least accurate, term which here is used only for changes not falling into the categories of dysplasia, *in situ* carcinoma or hyperplasia.

Dysplasia — A process of disordered cell growth which is used to describe changes at a cytologic level indicative of neoplastic transformation. It is used in this context here. The change may or may not be reversible. It is also recognized that similar cytologic changes may be the result of an inflammatory process and are reversible. Where this is apparent the term will always be qualified as inflammatory dysplasia.

In situ carcinoma — The severest form of dysplasia, still limited to the colonic mucosa, and as far as is known, having no metastatic potential. By definition, however, it also includes any mucosa from which invasive carcinoma is arising. In ulcerative colitis this is frequently less than the full picture of very severe dysplasia. However, this term will be used in the former context only.

Hyperplasia — Literally an increase in the number of cells. However, in ulcerative colitis this term has been applied to a change at the mildest end of the dysplasia spectrum characterized by moderately enlarged hyperchromatic nuclei pointing to the crypt lumen and in which it is uncertain whether the mild dysplasia is early neoplastic or postinflammatory. It is usually the latter. The increase in number of nuclei is probably only apparent and secondary to their undue prominence. The term is useful clinically to describe a mild change not having the sinister overtones of the word dysplasia and useful pathologically because there is no suitable alternative to accurately describe enlarged hyperchromatic nuclei other than those already defined above.

Invasive carcinoma — An infiltrative epithelial tumor which is no longer confined to the mucosa but has penetrated the muscularis mucosae and is, therefore, capable of metastasis.

Polyp — Any lesion projecting into the lumen of a hollow viscus and without any pathologic implication. Qualified variants include: 1) Adenomatous polyp — an intramucosal benign neoplastic epithelial tumor, 2) Inflammatory polyp — tags of normal or inflamed mucosa resulting from previous inflammation, and 3) "Pseudo" polyp — a nonpathological synonym for inflammatory polyp (definitely not pseudo).

THE PRECARCINOMATOUS LESION
MACROSCOPIC APPEARANCE

FLAT MUCOSA

Dysplasia frequently occurs in mucosa showing no distinguishing features from those usually seen in long-standing ulcerative colitis. The only possible recognition clinically is in patients who have a thickened or hyperplastic mucosa causing the usual atrophic appearance to become less easily recognized or to even disappear (Fig. 2). It is also possible that the submucosal vessels which are usually easy to see in ulcerative colitis might be difficult to see or be invisible under these circumstances. The lack of atrophy and indistinct submucosal vessels may, therefore, be a guide to which areas to biopsy, but no more than that.

VILLOUS MUCOSA

This change in the absence of an underlying carcinoma is recognizable in surgical specimens which have been opened, pinned out, and fixed as an area with an indistinct, slightly verrucose appearance because of the villi (Fig. 3). In the fresh specimen it has a somewhat velvety appearance and the villi vary from just visible on close inspection to readily visible, depending largely on size. Endoscopically this is more difficult to recognize, as viewing is necessarily carried out end-on rather than by direct vision from above. However, it is occasionally recognized by clinicians as a questionable villous tumor from which a biopsy is taken. The recognition of this lesion will clearly be facilitated by a wider knowledge of its existence.

POLYPOID MUCOSA

This is readily recognized in fresh and fixed specimens as well as endoscopically. However, there may be difficulty in distinquishing some inflammatory polyps from an adenoma, and this has been shown to be a spectrum.[1] As the

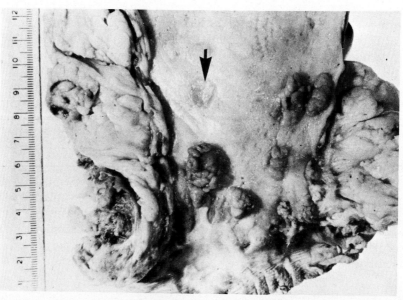

FIG. 2. Polypoid and flat precarcinomatous change and plaque-like carcinoma. Several discrete polypoid lesions are present, one being only slightly elevated above the surrounding mucosa. The intervening mucosa is opaque because of its increased thickness. A small plaque-like carcinoma is also present (arrow).

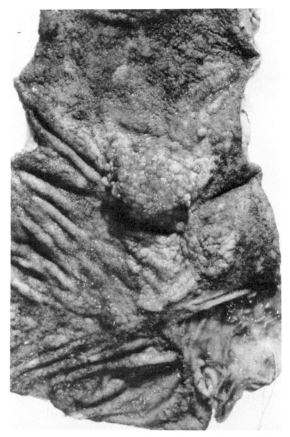

FIG. 3. Villous precarcinomatous change and nodular carcinoma. The specimen consists of terminal ileum (bottom right), cecum, and ascending colon. The nodule at the center is a small carcinoma. The surrounding mucosa is irregular and has a somewhat verrucose appearance, seen particularly at the top. Beneath the tumor the mucosa is rather more nodular.

incidence of invasive carcinoma in adenomas is closely related to size,[5] it is clearly advisable to excise endoscopically any polyp in which the head is 1 cm. or more in diameter (Fig. 2).

MICROSCOPIC APPEARANCE

Adenomatous formation and basal cell proliferation are commonly encountered changes; *in situ* anaplasia, clear cell transformation, and pancellular dysplasia are rarely encountered changes.

ADENOMATOUS CHANGE

This is the classical picture of neoplastic epithelium and occurs in flat, villous, and polypoid mucosa. When villi are present they may vary from rather broad to tall and slender structures (Fig 4.). Sometimes the villi have small tubules budding into their substance and this may produce club-shaped villi. In most villi the greatest dysplasia is usually seen at the base of the crypts and there is evidence of maturation as the top of the villus is approached. When club-shaped villi are present the reverse is frequently the case. As the villi decrease in height there is a greater tendency for them to bud, and this may be sufficiently marked to give rise to a back-to-back appearance.

A further feature discernible at low power is the amount of mucus present which tends to vary inversely with the amount of dysplasia, although this is not always the case. In areas of severe cytologic atypia there is usually no mucin production and the cytoplasm is eosinophilic (Fig. 5). Only an occasional goblet cell, or sometimes a minute amount of mucin in a very regular pattern on the luminal aspect of the cells, can just be discerned. When dysplasia is less marked there may be moderate amounts of mucin present. Goblet cells may appear normal but sometimes a regular row of goblet cells is present in which the mucous droplet occupies only about half of the cell (Fig. 6A). When dysplasia is mild there is frequently a normal or even an excessive amount of mucus (Fig. 6B); the cells often appear abnormally large and sometimes the goblet cells lose their polarity. Then the whole cell migrates towards the luminal surface and may be poorly oriented so that the nucleus is not on the basal side of the cell. Under these circumstances the cells usually become rounded and take on an appearance resembling signet ring cells.

Cell size is uniform although minor variations may be seen, particularly towards the tips of villi. The nuclei show all the characteristic features associated with neoplasia. They are usually rather uniformly hyperchromatic and elongated and it is difficult to see any nuclear detail. Occasional small nucleoli may be visible. Sometimes the nuclei are more vesicular with a heavy hyperchromatic peripheral chromatin rim and one or two nucleoli which are sometimes very prominent.

In the polypoid type of dysplasia there may be difficulty in the early stages distinguishing a true adenoma from a dysplastic inflammatory polyp (Fig. 7)

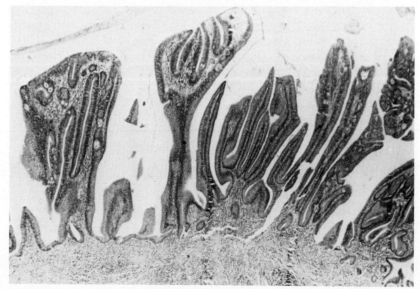

Fig. 4. Adenomatous change of villous type. Some villi are thin and slender, but in others budding of tubules at the tips has produced club-shaped villi. Hematoxylin and eosin; × 48.

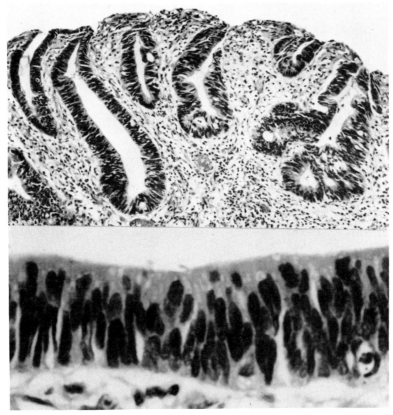

FIG. 5. Upper, severe adenomatous dysplasia (flat mucosa). Typical features of dysplasia are present. On the right, budding of tubules has produced a back-to-back arrangement of the crypts. Hematoxylin and eosin; × 190. Lower: High power showing the increased number of hyperchromatic nuclei with marked loss of polarity. Note the lack of goblet cells which produce a continuous well demarcated border to the cells. Hematoxylin and eosin; × 750.

and in the late stages it is impossible. While this appears to be semantics it is feasible to treat a solitary adenoma in the absence of dysplasia in the adjacent mucosa by simple polypectomy. However, the presence of numerous inflammatory polyps, several of which show dysplasia, suggests that a more generalized change is occurring and a more radical surgical procedure should be seriously considered.

While the adenomatous type of change has been described as occurring in flat, villous, and polypoid mucosa, carcinoma occurring in a flat mucosa is rare and there is usually transformation to a villous or more polypoid form in the immediate vicinity of the carcinoma.

Early adenomatous change is invariably found at the base of the crypts particularly when these are bifid (Fig. 6B). Rarely the luminal surface appears most dysplastic although this is more commonly seen in the early stages of the basal cell type of dysplasia. Figure 6 is probably the earliest lesion that can be considered to have invasive potential, although carcinoma seldom arises in a mucosa showing so little dysplasia. When carcinomas do arise from this type of

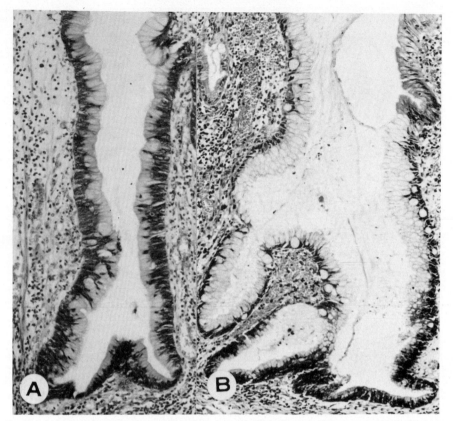

FIG. 6. *A*, moderate adenomatous dysplasia. Nuclei are enlarged and hyperchromatic but there is little loss of polarity and all the cells are mucus-producing. Hematoxylin and eosin; × 120. *B*, Mild adenomatous dysplasia which is limited to the base of the crypts. Marked crypt distortion and branching is present. In some goblet cells the mucus has become trapped and the cells rounded so that they resemble signet ring cells. Hematoxylin and eosin; × 120.

mucosa they are usually colloid cancers, and the epithelium lining the colloid vacuoles similarly shows surprisingly little dysplasia. Furthermore, these tumors may destroy the muscularis propria by an erosive process, so that the luminal surface rests directly on the remnants, if any, of the muscularis propria. Biopsies of these lesions may be very difficult to diagnose as carcinoma and this may only become apparent when the resected specimen is examined.

In some biopsies dysplasia is insufficiently severe to classify as early neoplastic and yet is out of proportion to that expected as a response to inflammation even when the inflammation present is taken into account. The only logical recourse in these circumstances is to request repeat biopsies.

BASAL CELL PROLIFERATION

This is most frequently seen in flat featureless mucosa where it occurs in a relatively pure form, but is often mixed with the adenomatous type of dysplasia especially in the polypoid form and more rarely in the villous form. It can arise in mucosa of normal or increased thicknesses. Cell size is often normal or only

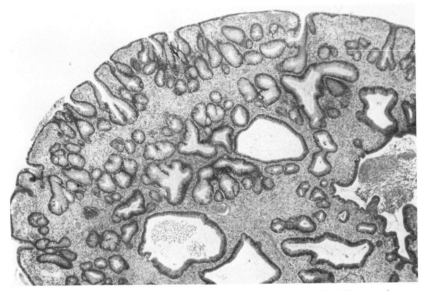

FIG. 7. Adenoma with mild dysplasia of dysplastic inflammatory polyp? The poorly organized array of crypts and lamina propria suggests that this may have been an inflammatory polyp. However, true adenoma in noncolitic patients can be similar. Hematoxylin and eosin; × 30.

moderately increased and the characteristic feature is a row of distinct, small, intensely hyperchromatic nuclei arranged linearly along the base of the cell (Fig. 8). The lack of the typical features of neoplasia including pleomorphism, loss of polarity, and nuclear crowding is typical and the appearance is not dissimilar to Beluga caviar arranged in a row (Fig. 9A). Occasional nuclei are slightly vesicular with a dense peripheral chromatin ring, a prominent nucleolus, mild pleomorphism but marked polychromatism (Fig 9B). The cytoplasm is similarly distinct and is usually markedly eosinophilic to the point of looking almost oncocytic. Furthermore, an identical appearance is seen throughout the whole length of the tubule, suggesting failure of cellular maturation. Goblet cells are absent. Sometimes evidence of maturation is seen as judged by the formation of goblet cells or a small row of mucin droplets close to the luminal border of the cell (Fig. 10). Mitotic activity is usually readily visible, at times it is intense, and mitotic figures can sometimes be found in the upper third of the crypts. Frequently, argentaffin, other clear cells, and Paneth cells may also be found. Inflammatory changes in the lamina propria are usually mild. The impression is that the cells at the base of the crypts pass to the surface with very little or no evidence of maturation, and it is for this reason that the term basal cell proliferation was chosen.

This is a particularly perplexing lesion, as it is difficult to believe from its appearance that it has any neoplastic potential. However, it appears to give rise directly to some of the very poorly differentiated tumors that characterize ulcerative colitis. The uniform appearance of both nucleus and cytoplasm along the crypt suggest that the cells are failing to mature as they progress towards the surface. When associated with a high mitotic index this might be because the turnover time is insufficient for the cells to mature as in subtotal villous

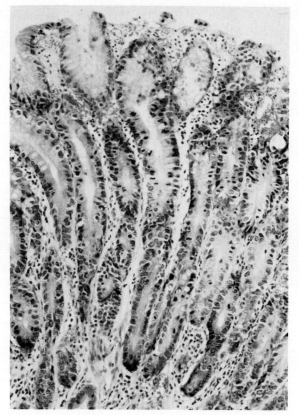

FIG. 8. Basal cell dysplasia. The low power appearance may be deceptively unimpressive and a thickened mucosa or closely packed crypts (as here) instead of the expected atrophy may be the only clue. Except for the cells in mitosis there is virtually no loss of polarity. Only an occasional goblet cell is present in the upper parts of the crypts. Hematoxylin and eosin; × 120.

atrophy in the jejunum, but when this is not apparent it is possible that the cells just fail to mature. The possibility that these cells are all absorptive cells with primary failure of goblet cell formation has to be considered but the nuclei are not the small rather vesicular normochromatic nuclei with small nucleoli that are typical of these cells. Furthermore, in many instances features of goblet cells can be discerned (Fig. 10.).

There may be considerable difficulty in identifying the early phase of basal cell proliferation as it is only with experience and awareness that the late stage is identified. Nevertheless, once the late lesion can be recognized, it becomes much easier to recognize the early stages which in their own way are also characteristic. The most noticeable feature is that only part of the crypt is involved, but because the lesion probably reflects a failure of maturation it is most readily identified in the luminal portions of the crypt where the lack of goblet cells and glassy eosinophilic cytoplasm are seen (Fig. 10, *right*, and Fig. 11). However, mitotic figures are not usually present while the characteristic nuclear changes are present but less well developed. Sometimes the changes are more obvious in the basal two-thirds of the crypts.

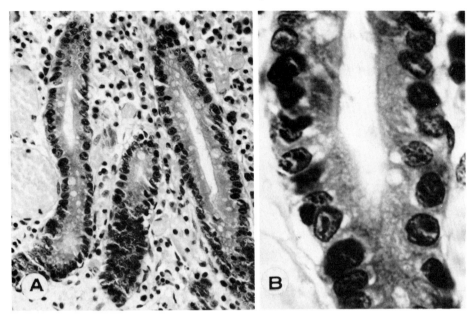

FIG. 9. *A*, basal cell dysplasia. The nuclei are distinct and most are hyperchromatic but there is variation in the intensity of nuclear staining. Note the absence of loss of polarity. The nuclei produce an appearance resembling a row of Beluga caviar. The sparsity of goblet cells produce a distinct inner border to the crypts and the cell cytoplasm is intensely eosinophilic. Hematoxylin and eosin; × 300. *B*, basal cell dysplasia. High power shows a surprising degree of nuclear pleomorphism and polychromatism despite the cells retaining their polarity. There is little tendency for the nuclei to overlap and nucleoli are variable in number and size. Hematoxylin and eosin; × 1200.

IN SITU ANAPLASIA

This is rare and has only been seen in flat mucosa. When present it is frequently associated with the basal cell type of dysplasia in the adjacent mucosa. It takes one of two forms. In one there is virtually no residual crypt structure but the mucosa consists of a sheet of small undifferentiated cells in which signet ring cells can usually be seen and sometimes may predominate. Surprisingly, in spite of the appearance this is often confined by the muscularis mucosa. The appearances resemble superficial spreading gastric carcinoma. However, once it becomes invasive, lymphatic and blood vessel permeation is easy to find.

In the second variety the crypt structure can still be discerned but the crypts appear to be breaking down. This form is even more uncommon that the first. In all cases examined there was little excess inflammation in the adjoining mucosa.

CLEAR CELL CHANGE

This is a further type of change which at first demands little attention because of its apparently innocuous appearance. It occurs as a slightly raised plaque and is characterised by large cells which are clear or have a faint ground glass appearance. The nuclei are elongated and hyperchromatic and there is some loss

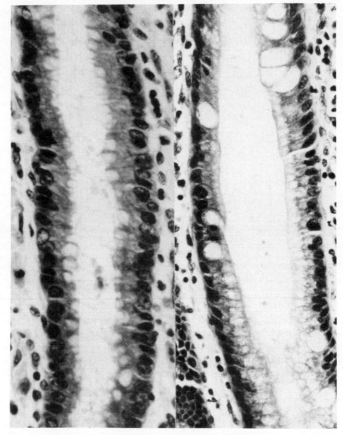

FIG. 10. Earlier basal cell dysplasia. Left, nuclei remain distinct and hyperchromatic but a row of mucus droplets are present on the luminal margin. Hematoxylin and eosin; × 480. Right, mild changes. Note the increase in mucus and occasional atypical goblet cells. The distinct nuclei are already apparent. Hematoxylin and eosin; × 300.

of polarity (Fig. 12). Occasional villi may be present. Carcinomas arising from this mucosa tend to be well differentiated. Close to the surface the lumen takes on an irregular arrangement that is reminiscent of the saw-toothed arrangement seen in metaplastic (hyperplastic) polyps. Paneth and argentaffin cells are not seen and mitotic figures are rare.

Pancellular Dysplasia

This is seen in flat featureless mucosa and is characterised by dysplasia which is manifest mainly as large hyperchromatic nuclei with loss of polarity. The change affects all cell lines including Paneth, argentaffin, and goblet cells. Paneth cells are prominent, are found away from their usual position at the base of the crypts, and appear to migrate up the crypt. Their nuclei lose their polarity and may be situated on the luminal side of the granules. Goblet cells tend to be distended with mucus, possibly an indication of an abnormality in the normal release mechanism. When the nucleus loses its polarity and appears as a crescent at the luminal border to the cell the comparison with a signet ring cell

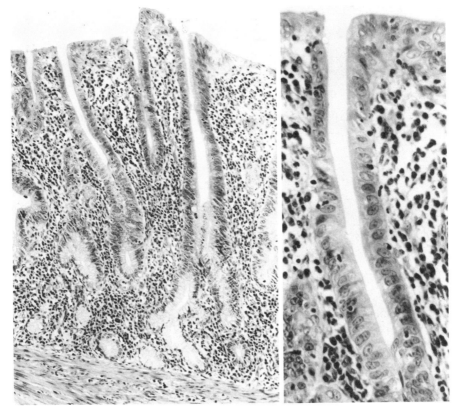

FIG. 11. Early basal cell dysplasia. Left, this usually begins in the upper portion of the crypts which fail to mature. The distinct crypt border and lack of goblet cells is apparent. The basal portion of the crypts show pseudopyloric metaplasia but this may be seen in any long-standing chronic inflammatory condition. Hematoxylin and eosin; × 120. Right, high power showing the distinct basally situated nuclei and lack of goblet cells. In this stage nuclei stain fairly uniformly. Hematoxylin and eosin; × 480.

seems unavoidable, although it may well be totally inappropriate. Argentaffin cells also appear far more numerous and may entirely surround the crypt giving an appearance resembling an *in situ* argentaffinoma. Any of these types of cells may predominate, but the other cell lines are invariably affected, albeit to a lesser degree.

THE PROBLEM OF EXPERIENCE

The great difficulty that the practicing pathologist will experience is the relative rarity with which these changes will be encountered in biopsies at any single institution. However, there are several methods that the pathologist can use to familiarize himself with these changes.

First, he can examine material in his files from patients with carcinoma complicating ulcerative colitis, and should he receive such a specimen, pay particular attention to the adjacent mucosa as well as the tumor. Most of these specimens contain a vast range of changes, and it is only by making the best use of these that the more subtle changes will become apparent.

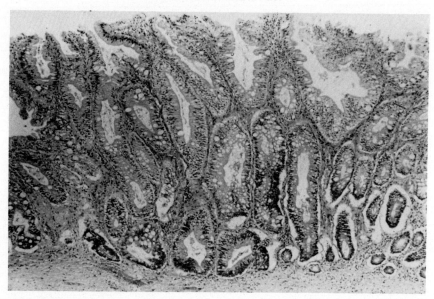

FIG. 12. Clear cell dysplasia. At first site there is a slight resemblance to a hyperplastic polyp with hyperchromatic nuclei particularly in the basal portion of the mucosa while in the superficial portion there is a suggestion of a saw-toothed pattern. The lumina are distinct with few goblet cells but the nuclei are enlarged and show more typical features of dysplasia. Hematoxylin and eosin; × 75.

Secondly, the pathologist must remain familiar with the wide spectrum of features that are seen in ulcerative colitis. To this end the clinician can be of value by providing regular biopsies from his colitic patients. It is virtually impossible for a pathologist to diagnose dysplasia unless absolutely obvious if he only receives a few rectal biopsies annually from colitic patients.

Finally, the importance of having a slide containing well oriented mucosa cannot be overemphasized. This is easily accomplished with rectal biopsies by treating them in a similar fashion to jejunal biopsies and mounting biopsies on any surface to prevent their curling. Once fixed, they are embedded on edge in paraffin and the sections that are cut will show the crypts in longitudinal section. In this way, the changes in various parts of the crypt can be studied.

Colonoscopic biopsies can prove more of a problem, but if biopsy forceps with a central spike are used the piece of mucosa obtained is already oriented within the biopsy cups, the submucosal surface being against the spike and the luminal surface against the cups. If the biopsy is scraped from the spike onto a flat surface, it should be oriented with luminal surface uppermost and can again be processed on edge. Sometimes it helps to mount the specimen on thin filter paper and to process the paper and specimen together, and this prevents loss of orientation during embedding. It is obvious that for good, well oriented biopsies to be obtained the cooperation of the clinician is required.

From these considerations it is apparent that the patients at risk are dependent on the cooperation of both the physician and pathologist if this tragic complication of ulcerative colitis is to be avoided. This can only be achieved if both are aware of each other's problems and combine to reduce these to a minimum.

ACKNOWLEDGMENTS

I am grateful to Dr. B. C. Morson for his advice and encouragement during this work which was carried out at St. Mark's Hospital, London, to Mr. Craig Rosner for the photographs, and to Ms. Betsy Hunt for her secretarial assistance.

REFERENCES

1. Dawson, I. M. P., and Pryse-Davies, J.: The development of carcinoma of the large intestine in ulcerative colitis. *Br. J. Surg. 47:* 113–128, 1959.
2. Devroede, G. J., Taylor, W. F., Sauer, W. G., Jackman, R. J., and Stickler, G. B.: Cancer risk and life expectancy of children with ulcerative colitis. *N. Engl. J. Med. 285:* 17–21, 1971.
3. Edwards, F. C., and Truelove, S. C.: The course and prognosis of ulcerative colitis. In *Carcinoma of the Colon,* Part IV. *Gut, 5:* 15–22 1964.
4. Hultén, L., Kewenter, J., and Ahrén, C.: Precancer and carcinoma in chronic ulcerative colitis; a histopathological and clinical investigation. *Scand. J. Gastroenterol. 7:* 663–669, 1972.
5. Muto, T., Bussey, H. J. R., and Morson, B. C.: The polyp-cancer sequence in the large bowel. *Proc. R. Soc. Med. 67:* 451–457, 1974.
6. Morson, B. C., and Pang, L. S. C.: Rectal biopsy as an aid to cancer control in ulcerative colitis. *Gut 8:* 423–434, 1967.
7. Mottet, N. K.: Histopathologic spectrum of regional enteritis and ulcerative colitis. In *Major Problems in Pathology,* vol. II. Toronto, W. B. Saunders, 1971.
8. Myrvold, H. E., Kock, N. G., Ahrén, C.: Rectal biopsy and precancer in ulcerative colitis. *Gut 15:* 301–304, 1974.
9. Yardley, J. H., Keren, D. F.: "Precancer" lesions in ulcerative colitis: A retrospective study of rectal biopsy and colectomy specimens. *Cancer 34:* 835–844, 1974.

Chapter 9

The Etiology of Colonic Cancer*

M. J. HILL

Although there are still some dissenters,[16] it is generally accepted that large bowel cancer has a dietary etiology. There is no agreement on the responsible dietary component (Table 1); correlations based on international statistical data suggest fat, animal protein, or meat[3, 15, 18, 37] while comparisons of Africans and western peoples have led to the incrimination of refined carbohydrate and fiber depletion.[7, 33] Case control studies have implicated fat,[35] meat, and particularly beef,[19] crude fiber,[30] and some vitamins.[4] All of these dietary items have their supporters and the evidence in favor of any one of them is certainly inadequate to win converts. I have already stated my reasons for believing that fat is the most important dietary item in the causation of this disease,[23] and for believing that fiber plays no causative role.

Because the search for a dietary carcinogen to explain the disease has not proved successful, a group of us have been working since 1967[6] on the postulate that the carcinogen is produced *in situ* in the large bowel by bacterial action either on a dietary component or on some secretion produced in response to the diet.

INITIAL INVESTIGATIONS OF THE POSTULATE

We chose as our postulated substrate the bile acids. Initial studies on two populations[1, 2] showed that people living in Uganda, where the incidence of large bowel cancer is low, have a lower fecal bile acid concentration, less bacterially degraded bile acids, and fewer nonsporing anaerobic bacteria in their feces than people living in London where the incidence of large bowel cancer is moderately high. In view of this success the study was extended to 6[27] and later to 9 populations[26] with equally favorable results, and these findings were subsequently confirmed in another laboratory.[36]

The next step was to select from within a country a number of populations with different incidences of large bowel cancer but similar in as many other respects as possible. In Hong Kong people with relatively high incomes eat a diet which is much richer in meat and fat than that of the lower income groups. We found that the high income population had a higher fecal bile acid concentration than the low income group by a factor of more than 2;[24] a recent epidemio-

* This work is supported financially by the Cancer Research Campaign.

logic study has shown that the incidence of large bowel cancer is greater by a very similar factor in the high income group.[12]

Thus, our early data supported the postulate that large bowel cancer is caused by a bacterial metabolite of bile acids. The next problem was to determine the nature of the metabolite. Initially we suggest that the bacteria produced a fully aromatic metabolite;[22] this would theoretically need only four types of reaction and we have demonstrated all four using gut bacteria.[26] In three of these the bacteria carrying out the reaction were lecithinase-negative clostridia which produced butyric acid from glucose fermentation, and preliminary studies showed that these organisms were more numerous in the feces of people living in countries with a high incidence of large bowel cancer than in those with a low incidence of the disease.[17] On reflection we have abandoned the concept of a polycyclic aromatic metabolite and now favor the postulate that bile acids with only one or two double bonds are the metabolites important in large bowel cancer,[25] and that they act as co-carcinogens rather than as complete carcinogens. Hofmann and his co-workers have demonstrated that such nuclear dehydrogenation reactions take place in the human gut.[21]

Our next step was to embark on a case-comparison study in collaboration with clinicians at St. Mark's Hospital and Northwick Park Hospital. In this study the stools of persons entering the gastroenterology wards of the two hospitals were analyzed for fecal bile acid concentration (FBA) and for the presence of clostridia able to dehydrogenate the bile acid nucleus (NDC). If our postulate is correct then the requirements for optimal production of co-carcinogen are a combination of high FBA and the presence of NDC. Of 93 patients with gastrointestinal disease other than large bowel cancer 8 had this combination, compared with 31 of 44 large bowel cancer patients.[28] This latter group has now been extended to more than 100 and these have been subdivided into roughly similar numbers of colonic and rectal carcinomas. The proportion of each group with the high risk conbination of FBA and NDC was similar for both groups (Table 2). Subdivision of the rectum into three parts revealed that the proportion with the combination was similar for all three subdivisions. Haenszel and Correa[20] have suggested on the basis of epidemiologic data that carcinoma of the lower rectum has a different etiology from that of other colorectal cancers. A relatively low proportion of persons with carcinoma of the cecum and ascending colon had the high risk combination of fecal analyses and although the number of patients in this

TABLE 1. DIETARY FACTORS IMPLICATED IN THE ETIOLOGY OF LARGE BOWEL CANCER

Dietary item	Type of study	Reference
Fat	International correlation	15, 37
	Case-control study	35
Animal protein	International correlation	18
Meat	International correlation	3
	Case-control study	19
Fiber depletion	Comparison; Africa vs. "the west"	7
	Comparison of populations within South Africa	33
	Case-control study	30
Vitamins	Case-control study	4

group is small the results are in agreement with the suggestion by Haenszel and Correa[20] that right-sided and left-sided tumors have different etiologies.

CURRENT STUDIES

Because the results to date have been so encouraging we have now embarked on a series of prospective studies (Table 3). These include: 1) a study of 10,000 normal persons aged 45 to 75 years, 2) a study of patients who have had chronic ulcerative colitis with total involvement for more than 10 years, 3) a study of persons who have had a primary large bowel carcinoma removed by resection, and 4) a study of persons with familial polyposis and their offspring and siblings. Of these, the study of normal persons is by far the most important but is also the most long-term. It is being carried out in collaboration with physicians in three general practices (Dr. J. Hart and his partners in Glycorrwg, a mining village in S. Wales; Dr. D. Wilson and his partners in Hay-on-Wye, a farming area in Herefordshire; and of Dr. E. Kuenssberg and his partners in the old dockland area of Edinburgh), with Dr. T. W. Meade and his colleagues in the epidemiology department of Northwick Park Hospital, and with the Medical Research Council (MRC) Nutrition Unit at Cambridge. In all, 10,000 persons aged 45 to 75 years will be recruited into the study and they will contribute a stool sample and

TABLE 2. PROPORTION OF PATIENTS WITH THE COMBINATION OF HIGH FBA[a] AND HIGH NDC[b] IN RELATION TO THE SITE OF THE TUMOR

Site of the tumor	No. of patients	% with high FBA[a] and NDC[b]
Colon	40	73
Cecum and ascending and transverse	11	45
Descending and sigmoid	29	83
Rectum	67	75
Upper	17	76
Mid	15	73
Lower	20	80
Unassigned	15	67

[a] FBA = fecal bile acid concentration.
[b] NDC = clostridia able to dehydrogenate the bile acid nucleus.

TABLE 3. A SUMMARY OF THE GROUPS TO BE STUDIED PROSPECTIVELY TO TEST THE VALUE OF THE COMBINATION OF HIGH FBA AND NDC AS AN INDICATOR OF RISK OF DEVELOPING LARGE BOWEL CANCER

Group studied	No. of persons in the group	No. recruited to date	No. of cancer cases expected by 1980
A. Normal healthy persons aged 45–75 years	10,000	3,000	50–100
B. Patients with ulcerative colitis with total involvement for more than 10 years	100–150	80	10–20
C. Patients who have had a large bowel carcinoma resected			
(a) adenoma present at resection	200	80	20–30 ?
(b) no adenoma present at resection	200	150	5–10 ?
D. Patients with familial polyposis (F.P.)	30	12	
their siblings	100	60	50 (as F.P.)

Studies B, C, and D are in collaboration with Dr. B. Morson, Dr. R. Bussey, and the clinicians at St. Mark's Hospital, London, while A is a multi-center study.

fill in a short questionnaire concerning bowel habits, use of laxatives etc., and previous abdominal surgery. In addition we hope to carry out a diet survey of the population and to measure intestinal transit times. In such a study it is important to get as high a proportion as possible of the persons in the relevant age group into the study, and this is largely an exercise in public relations and pre-publicity. We have faith in the value of the study and in our ability to persuade the general public of this value. To date, more than 75% of those asked have cooperated fully in the study despite the fact that we stress that this will be of no benefit to them personally. We hope to have meaningful results in about 5 years, but will continue the follow up for about 10 years, primarily through the general practitioners, the Cancer Registries, and the Central Records Department at Southport. The stool analyses of those who develop large bowel cancer will be compared with those of persons who die of other diseases.

The investigations of the high risk patient groups will give answers more quickly but the interpretation of the results may be more difficult. All three groups of high risk patients are being studied in collaboration with St. Mark's Hospital. Patients who have had chronic ulcerative colitis with total colonic involvement for more than 10 years have a high risk of developing large bowel cancer.[29, 31] There are more than 100 such patients who attend the outpatient clinic of St. Mark's Hospital regularly for routine examinations and rectal biopsy for precancerous change. It is possible that these patients are at high risk of developing large bowel cancer simply because the colonic mucosa is permanently inflamed and consequently more sensitive to any carcinogens present in the luminal contents. The difference between those who develop large bowel cancer and those who do not might merely reflect differences in sensitivity to a fairly equal carcinogen load. Alternatively, although the colonic tissue is undoubtedly more exposed than in the normal healthy person the exposure may be about equal in all of these patients and the difference between those who develop carcinoma and those who do not would then reflect differences in carcinogen load that we could hope to detect from the fecal analyses. Already two of the patients have developed severe dysplasia and a third had developed large bowel cancer; all three would be judged to be at very high risk by the criteria of the fecal analyses. These are very preliminary results, but if they are confirmed they will indicate that the cancer is due to increased carcinogen load rather than to increased sensitivity, and also that our analyses provide an index of that increased carcinogen level.

Patients who have had a primary large bowel carcinoma resected successfully are at high risk of developing a second primary large bowel carcinoma. Consequently we can look for the proportion of people in this group of patients with our high risk combination of FBA and NDC compared with the normal population. Preliminary studies indicate that 25% of these patients have the high risk combination, indicating a risk of developing large bowel cancer 3 times that in the normal population. Because of the relatively small size of the study group it is difficult to estimate with certainty the true excess risk in this population but Polk *et al.*[32] have suggested that nearly a third of such patients will develop a further large bowel carcinoma, about 6 times that of the population as a whole. Analysis of the data at St. Mark's Hospital indicates that those persons in whom there was one or more adenomas at the time of excision of the carcinoma are at much higher risk of developing a subsequent second primary large bowel tumor than are those in whom there were no adenomas.[9] Consequently we are dividing our patients into two groups dependent on the presence or absence of adenomas at the time of resection. The numbers of patients are, of course, small at present, but our analyses are in agreement with the epidemiologic findings at St. Mark's Hospital. Further, they suggest that in the absence of a concurrent adenoma the proportion of people with the high risk combination is no different from that in the normal population; it would be interesting to know whether or not this subgroup has any increased risk of a second primary large bowel carcinoma.

One obvious conclusion to be drawn from these studies is that, if before resection 75% have the high risk combination compared with only 25% after resection, the resection procedure is accompanied by a major change in fecal composition. In general we find that in a high proportion of these patients the fecal steroid concentration falls sharply following the operation (often by a factor of 4). The proportion is greater following resection of rectal than of colonic carcinomas. Unfortunately we do not have data on the daily fecal loss of bile acids and so we do not know whether this fall is due to a reduced amount of bile acid or to the presence of some diluting factor normally degraded in the complete large bowel; in the shortened bowel following resection the transit of material is more rapid[14] and so slowly degraded components would remain only partially digested.

The fourth group that we are studying consists of the persons with familial polyposis coli and their offspring. Since persons with this disease will certainly go on to develop large bowel cancer,[31] and since the carcinoma has an identical pathology to that in nonadenomatosis persons,[8] it has been suggested that these patients present an ideal opportunity to investigate the etiology of large bowel cancer. In collaboration with St. Mark's Hospital we have been studying the stools of patients with familial polyposis. We have also analysed the stools of the children of these patients, since about half of the children should go on to develop the disease.[8]

We have confirmed the findings of Core and Watne[11] that in these patients cholesterol is not reduced to coprostanol in the intestine: in the normal person 80 to 90% of the neutral steroids are in the form of the bacterial metabolites coprostanol and coprostanone. Further, the children of polyposis patients segregate into two groups[5] — those who excrete their neutral steroids as cholesterol (polyposis type) and those whose neutral steroids are mainly in the form of the bacterial metabolites (normal type). It will be interesting to see whether the children with polyposis type neutral steroids will go on to develop polyposis while those with normal fecal neutral steroids will be the unaffected siblings or whether this is of no value as an early indicator of the disease.

In our experience, the lack of cholesterol degradation in the gut found in the polyposis patients is rare in persons without this disease (Table 4), in contrast with the findings of Wilkins and Hackman.[34] The fecal flora isolated from the polyposis patients had a normal composition and was able to reduce cholesterol to coprostanol readily when tested *in vitro* by the method of Coleman and Baumann.[10] Thus the lack of cholesterol degradation in the gut must be due to adverse conditions rather than to any abnormality in the organisms *per se.* We therefore looked at other substrates and found that they, too, were not being metabolized to the usual extent; bile salts were not even being completely deconjugated, urinary cyclic secondary amines (produced from basic amino acids in the gut) were not detectable, and urinary phenols (formed in the gut by bacterial action on aromatic amino acids) were only produced in small amounts (Table 5). When tested *in vitro,* the fecal bacteria of polyposis patients have the normal ability to deconjugate and dehydroxylate bile acids and to metabolize the amino acids, and so the conditions must be unfavorable for bacterial metabolism in general, not just for cholesterol metabolism. To date we have looked at three factors that could be responsible for the lack of bacterial activity: the intestinal pH, E_h, and transit time. Transit time was measured by the method of Cummings[13] in three patients with familial polyposis and in all three it was in the normal range; fecal pH was measured in 6 polyposis patients and was in the normal range of between 6 and 7.5 in all; fecal E_h as indicated by the ratio of anaerobic to aerobic organisms in the faeces was also normal. In our studies of

TABLE 4. THE PROPORTIONS OF PERSONS IN VARIOUS POPULATIONS WITH A HIGH PROPORTION OF UNDEGRADED CHOLESTEROL IN THEIR STOOLS

Population	No. of persons studied	% In which cholesterol accounts for more than 75% of the neutral steroids
English		
Normal persons	56	0
Large bowel cancer patients	59	2
Patients with other gastrointestinal diseases (total)	43	4
Scottish[15]	15	0
English Vegans	15	0
United States		
White[15]	41	9
Black	12	0
Hong Kong	64	16
Japan	36	44
India	11	0
Uganda	11	9
South Africa		
Black	23	26
White	13	0
Finland	23	0
Denmark	21	0

TABLE 5. PRODUCTS OF BACTERIAL METABOLISM IN THE GUT OF NORMAL PERSONS AND OF PERSONS WITH FAMILIAL POLYPOSIS

	Normal persons	Patients with familial polyposis
Reduction of cholesterol to coprostanol (mg/day)	300–500	0–30
Monosubstituted bile acid (mg/day)	80–150	20–40
Metabolism of basic amino acids to cyclic secondary amines (mg/day)	500–1500	< 50
Metabolism of aromatic amino acids to volatile phenols (mg/day)	70–100	20–30

gut bacterial activity we have found that compounds are metabolized well unless the transit of the substrate through the gut is so rapid that the person had diarrhea; this was not so in any of our polyposis patients. Most of the gut bacterial enzymes that we have studied have pH optima between 6 and 7, and an acid stool often indicates a low level of bacterial activity in the gut, but this could not explain the lack of bacterial activity in the gut of polyposis patients. Most gut bacteria are strictly anaerobic and need cultural conditions that are highly anaerobic if they are to produce their full array of enzymes, but the conditions must have been highly reducing in the gut to permit the anaerobes to dominate the aerotolerant organisms so greatly. Lack of bacterial activity does not characterize all patients with multiple intestinal polyps, since patients with the Peutz-Jeghers syndrome have normal gut bacterial activity. At present, therefore, we have no explanation for the lack of bacterial activity in the gut of familial polyposis patients. We have only observed a similar phenomenon in volunteers fed a soluble, totally absorbable diet, and it is difficult to see how this can be related to the problem of polyposis.

CONCLUSIONS

Our study of patients with familial polyposis provides no support for our theory on the etiology of large bowel cancer. However, it is not surprising that in this disease the genetic component of its etiology so dominates the environmental. In contrast the early data from the study of patients with ulcerative colitis and of patients treated for a first primary large bowel carcinoma by resection and anastomosis provide a modicum of support for our postulate that large bowel cancer is caused by an unsaturated bile acid produced by bacterial action in the gut. The most crucial study, the prospective study in normal persons, is also the most long-term. If the results of that study should also support our postulate, then we will be in a position to attempt to reduce the incidence of this disease by the methods that we have discussed previously.[24]

ACKNOWLEDGMENTS

Of the persons working in this laboratory and actively participating in the studies described here I should particularly acknowledge the role of Dr. B. S. Drasar (who has been associated with this work from its inception) and also Mr. P. Borriello, Miss F. Fernandez, Mrs. S. Heaton, Mr. T. Jivraj, and Miss K. Johnson.

REFERENCES

1. Aries, V., Crowther, J. S., Drasar, B. S., and Hill, M. J.: Degradation of bile salts by human intestinal bacteria. *Gut 10:* 575–576, 1969.
2. Aries, V., Crowther, J. S., Drasar, B. S., Hill, M. J., and Williams, R. E. O.: Bacteria and the aetiology of cancer of the large bowel. *Gut 10:* 334–335, 1969.
3. Armstrong, B., and Doll, R.: Environmental factors and cancer incidence and mortality in different countries, with special reference to dietary practices. *Int. J. Cancer 15:* 617–631, 1975.
4. Bjelke, E. Epidemiological studies of cancer of the stomach, colon and rectum; with special emphasis on the role of diet. *Scand. J. Gastroenterol.* (Suppl. 31) *9:* 1–235, 1974.
5. Bone, E., Drasar, B. S., and Hill, M. J.: Gut bacteria and their metabolic activities in familial polyposis. *Lancet 1:* 1117–1120, 1975.
6. British Empire Cancer Campaign for Research. Forty-fifth annual Report covering the year 1967.

7. Burkitt, D. P.: Epidemiology of cancer of the colon and rectum. *Cancer 28:* 3-13, 1971.
8. Bussey, H. J. R.: *Familial Polyposis Coli: Family studies, histopathology, differential diagnosis and results of treatment.* Baltimore, The John Hopkins University Press, 1975.
9. Bussey, H. J. R., Wallace, M. H., and Morson, B. C.: Metachronous carcinoma of the large intestine and intestinal polyps. *Proc. R. Soc. Med. 60:* 208-210, 1967.
10. Coleman, D. L., and Baumann, C. A.: Intestinal sterols. V. Reduction of sterols by intestinal microorganisms. *Arch. Biochem. Biophys. 72:* 219-225, 1957.
11. Core, S. K., and Watne, A. L.: Fecal steroids and colon cancer (abstract). *Fed. Proc., 33:* 260, 1974.
12. Crowther, J. S., Drasar, B. S., Hill, M. J., Maclennan R., Magnin, D., Peach, S., and Teoh-Chan, C. H.: Faecal steroids and bacteria and large bowel cancer mortality in Hong Kong by socio-economic indicators. *Brit. J. Cancer 34:* 191-198, 1976.
13. Cummings, J. In preparation.
14. Cummings, J. H. James, W. P. T., and Wiggins, H. S.: Role of the colon in ileal-resection diarrhoea. *Lancet i:* 344-347, 1973.
15. Drasar, B. S. and Irving, D.: Environmental factors and cancer of the colon and breast. *Br. J. Cancer 27:* 167-172, 1973.
16. Enstrom, J. E.: Colorectal cancer and consumption of beef and fat. *Br. J. Cancer 32:* 432-439, 1975.
17. Goddard, P., Fernandez, F., West, B., Hill, M. J., and Barnes, P.: The nuclear dehydrogenation of steroids by intestinal bacteria. *J. Med. Microbiol. 8:* 429-435, 1975.
18. Gregor, O., Toman, R., and Prusova, F.: Gastrointestinal cancer and nutrition. *Gut 10:* 1031-1034, 1969.
19. Haenszel, W., Berg, J. W., Segi, M., Kurihara, M., and Locke, F. B.: Large bowel cancer in Hawaiian Japanese. *J. Natl. Cancer Inst. 51:* 1765-1779, 1973.
20. Haenszel, W., and Correa, P.: Cancer of the large intestine: Epidemiologic findings. *Dis. Colon Rectum 16:* 371-377, 1973.
21. Hepner, G. W., Hofmann, A. F., and Thomas, P. J.: Metabolism of steroid and amino acid moieties of conjugated bile acids in man. II. Glycine conjugated dihydroxyfile acids. *J. Clin. Invest. 51:* 1898-1905, 1972.
22. Hill, M. J.: In *Some Implications of Steroid Hormones in Cancer.* edited by Williams, D. C., and Briggs, M. H., p. 94. London, Heinemann, 1971.
23. Hill, M. J.: Colon cancer: A disease of fibre depletion or of dietary excess? *Digestion 11:* 289-306, 1974.
24. Hill, M. J.: Steroid nuclear dehydrogenation and colon cancer. *Am. J. Clin. Nutr. 27:* 1475-1480, 1974.
25. Hill, M. J.: The role of colon anaerobes in the metabolism of bile acids and steroids and its relation to colon cancer. *Cancer 36:* 2387-2400, 1975.
26. Hill, M. J., and Drasar, B. S.: Bacteria and the etiology of cancer of the large intestine. In *Anaerobic Bacterial: Role in Disease*, Ch. XII, edited by Balows, A., De Haan, R. M., Dowell, V. R., and Guze, L. B., pp. 119-133. Springfield, Charles C Thomas, 1974.
27. Hill, M. J., Drasar, B. S., Aries, V. C., Crowther, J. S., Hawksworth, G., and Williams, R. E. O.: Bacteria and aetiology of cancer of large bowel. *Lancet i:* 95-100, 1971.
28. Hill, M. J., Drasar, B. S., Williams, R. E. O., Meade, T. W., Cox, A. G., Simpson, J. E. P., and Morson, B. C.: Faecal bile acids and clostridia in patients with cancer of the large bowel. *Lancet i:* 535-538, 1975.
29. MacDougall, I. P. M.: Clinical identification of those cases of ulcerative colitis most likely to develop cancer of the bowel. *Dis. Colon Rectum 7:* 447-450, 1964.
30. Modan, B., Barell, V., Lubin, F., Modan, M., Greenberg, R. A., and Graham, S.: Low-fiber intake as an etiologic factor in cancer of the colon. *J. Natl. Cancer Inst. 55:* 15-18, 1975.
31. Morson, B. C., and Bussey, H. J. R.: Predisposing causes of intestinal cancer. In *Current Problems in Surgery.* Chicago, Year Book Medical Publishers, 1970.
32. Polk, H. C., Spratt, J. S. and Butcher, H. R.: Frequency of multiple primary malignant neoplasms associated with colorectal carcinoma. *Am. J. Surg. 109:* 71-75, 1965.
33. Walker, A. R. P.: Crude fibre, bowel motility and pattern of diet. *S. Afr. Med. J. 35:* 114-115, 1961.

34. Wilkins, T. D. and Hackman, A. S.: Two patterns of neutral steroid conversion in the feces of normal North Americans. *Cancer Res. 34:* 2250–2254, 1974.

35. Wynder, E. L., Kajitani, T., Ishikawa, S., Dodo, H., and Takano, A.: Environmental factors of cancer of the colon and rectum. II. Japanese epidemiological data. *Cancer 23:* 1210–1220, 1969.

36. Wynder, E. L., and Reddy, B. S.: Metabolic epidemiology of colorectal cancer. *Cancer 34:* 801–806, 1974.

37. Wynder, E. L., and Shigematsu, T.: Environmental factors of cancer of the colon and rectum. *Cancer 20:* 1520–1561, 1967.

Chapter 10

Prognostic Factors in Colon Carcinoma: Correlation of Serum Carcinoembryonic Antigen Level and Tumor Histopathology*,†

NORMAN ZAMCHECK, WILHELM G. DOOS, ROMULO PRUDENTE,
BENJAMIN B. LURIE, AND LEONARD S. GOTTLIEB

It is widely agreed that histopathologic grading of malignant tumors provides prognostically useful information.[20] Recent studies with carcinoembryonic antigen (CEA) have suggested that circulating levels of CEA may also be prognostically useful.[8, 40] Accordingly, the present study was designed to compare circulating CEA levels obtained before resection of colon cancer with the histopathology of the tumors and with the postoperative clinical course. In addition to grading by the Dukes and Broders techniques, the degree of lymphocytic and plasma cell infiltration of the tumor was graded and the extent of tumor invasion of lymphatic vessels, nerves, and blood vessels was correlated with circulating CEA levels. The prognostic significance of the tumor morphology was reinforced by the CEA findings.

MATERIALS AND METHODS

Forty-five specimens of primary colonic adenocarcinoma obtained at surgery were studied. The morphologic features were correlated with preoperative serum CEA levels.

Pathologic studies were done independently of clinical examination. Resected specimens were examined in the fresh state, opened along the antimesenteric border, and fixed in 10% formalin for 24 hours after being pinned to a flat surface with the mucosal surface up. Subsequently the tumor was examined in multiple sections, and samples were selected from the deepest point of tumor invasion and from the tumor periphery. Hematoxylin- and eosin-stained sections of the

* Study supported by National Cancer Institute grant CA-04486 and contract NIH-NCI NO1 CP 33264, National Institutes of Health, and by grant IM-18B from the American Cancer Society.
† Reprinted from: N. Zamcheck, W. G. Doos, R. Prudente, B. B. Lurie, and L. S. Gottlieb: Prognostic factors in colon carcinoma: correlation of serum carcinoembryonic antigen level and tumor histopathology. *Human Pathology 6:* 31–45, 1975, by permission of the publisher, W. B. Saunders Company.

colonic lesions were examined. The tumor was classified as Dukes A, B, or C on the basis of the depth of bowel wall penetration and regional lymph node metastasis[9, 10] and was also graded according to Broders I to IV scale of malignancy.[25] "Round cell" infiltration at the periphery of the advancing edges of the tumor was graded on a scale from 0 to 3+, the latter indicating extensive infiltration by either lymphocytes or plasma cells (Figs. 1 to 3). Areas of necrosis were avoided. Lymphatic, blood vessel, and perineural invasion was searched for (Figs. 4, 5). Lymphatic invasion was classified as "certain" when tumor cells were unequivocally present in lymphatic channels, as "suggestive" when tumor cells were observed in tissue clefts lined with endothelium, and as "presumptive" when metastases were noted in regional lymph nodes. The presence of vascular invasion was confirmed by elastic tissue stains when indicated.

Serum CEA assays were carried out in blind duplicate by the method of Thomson.[36] The preoperative CEA levels were not known until after the morphologic studies were completed, thus providing a "blind" and unbiased correlation of tumor morphology and the CEA level. The microscopic sections were reviewed by three pathologists who agreed essentially on the findings. For purposes of assessing prognosis the patients were clinically followed for an average of 17 months after resection (range, 3 to 32 months; Tables 1 and 2).

RESULTS

The results of histopathologic study, the CEA levels, and clinical data are presented in Table 1. Thirteen patients were classified as Dukes A, 11 as Dukes

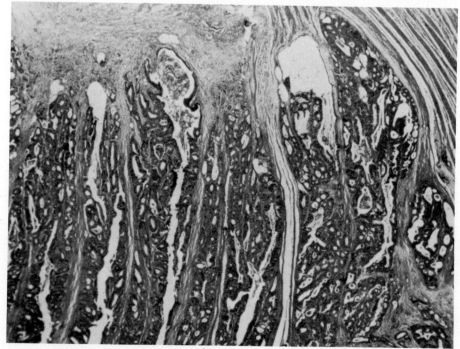

Fig. 1. Invading adenocarcinoma showing no infiltrate at the advancing edges of the tumor. Hematoxylin and eosin stain, × 10.

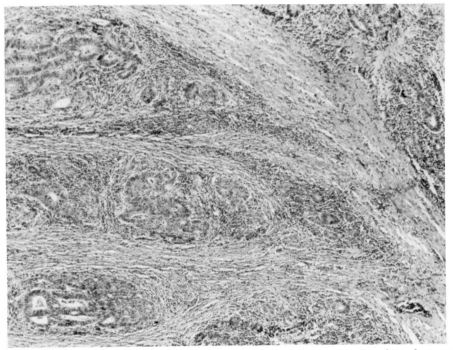

FIG. 2. Lymphocyte-plasma cell infiltrate regarded as 3+ at the advancing edges of a tumor. Hematoxylin and eosin stain, × 50.

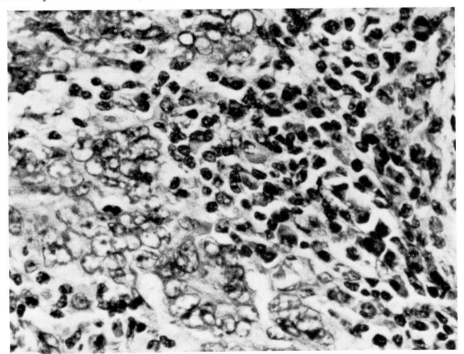

FIG. 3. High power view of infiltrate. Both plasma cells and lymphocytes are present. Hematoxylin and eosin stain, × 450.

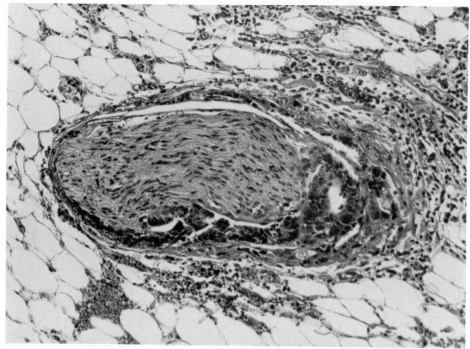

FIG. 4. Adenocarcinoma infiltrating perineural space. Hematoxylin and eosin stain, × 100.

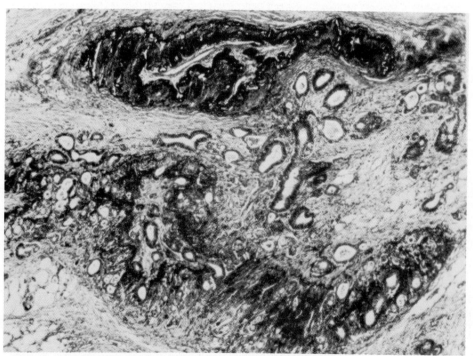

FIG. 5. Obliterated vein showing invasive adenocarcinoma. Verhoeff's elastic stain, × 50.

TABLE 1. HISTOLOGIC AND CLINICAL DATA IN 45 PATIENTS WITH COLONIC CARCINOMA

Case No.	Duration of Follow-up (Months)	Present Status*	Dukes Classification	Broders Classification	Round Cell Infiltrates*		Structural Invasion	CEA Titer (ng./ml.)
1	24	Well	B	II	L+	P0	0	< 1.0
2	22	Mets.	C	II	L0	P+	Lymph	3.1
3	12	Mets.	C	II	L0	P0	Lymph, vein, nerve	3.7
4	25	Mets.	C	II	L+	P0	Lymph	> 10.0
5	3	Exp., mets.	C	II	L0	P0	Lymph, vein	> 10.0
6	16	Well	B	II	L+	P++	0	< 1.0
7	24	Well	B	II	L0	P0	0	4.8
8	26	Well	A	II	L+	P+	0	< 1.0
9	10	Exp., mets.	C	II	L+	P+	Lymph	1.7
10	17	Well	A	II	L++	P++	0	< 1.0
11	28	Well	B	II	L++	P0	0	< 1.0
12	31	Well	A	I	L++	P++	0	< 1.0
13	27	Mets.	B	III	L0	P0	Lymph, vein	< 1.0
14	—	Uncertain	A	I	L++	P++	0	1.4
15	18	Well	A	I	L+++	P+	0	< 1.0
16	22	Well	B	II	L++	P++	0	2.3
17	7	Exp.†	A	II	L+	P0	0	2.4
18	22	Well	B	II	L0	P0	Lymph	3.7
19	9	Well	C	II	L+	P0	Lymph	2.9
20	25	Well	A	II	L+	P+	0	< 1.0
21	8	Exp., mets.	A	I	L++	P0	0	< 1.0
22	5	Well	A	I	L+	P++	0	< 1.0
23	29	Well	A	III	L+	P0	0	4.2
24	4	Exp., mets.	C	IV	L0	P0	Lymph, vein	> 10.0
25	—	Uncertain	C	III	L0	P0	Lymph	> 10.0
26	28	Mets.	C	II	L0	P0	Lymph, vein, nerve	7.6
27	12	Mets.	C	II	L0	P0	Lymph, vein	> 10.0
28	8	Well	C	II	L++	P++	Lymph	1.7
29	13	Well	A	I	L++	P++	0	< 1.0
30	10	Well	C	II	L+	P+++	Lymph	2.7
31	8	Well	C	II	L0	P0	Lymph	> 10.0
32	24	Well	B	II	L+	P+	Lymph	2.8
33	16	Well	B	II	L+	P0	0	< 1.0
34	19	Well	B	II	L+	P0	0	6.2
35	12	Well	C	III	L++	P++	Lymph	> 10.0
36	14	Exp., mets.	C	IV	L0	P0	Lymph, vein, nerve	> 10.0
37	9	Well	B	II	L+	P++	0	1.0
38	14	Well	A	II	L+	P0	0	< 1.0
39	17	Mets.	C	II	L+	P0	Lymph	2.5
40	26	Well	A	I	L++	P0	0	2.1
41	8	Exp., mets.	C	III	L0	P0	Lymph	> 10.0
42	—	Uncertain	C	II	L+	P0	Lymph	> 10.0
43	24	Mets.	C	II	L0	P0	Lymph	> 10.0
44	8	Exp.†	C	II	L+	P0	Lymph, nerve	> 10.0
45	20	Mets.	C	II	L0	P0	Lymph, vein	> 10.0

*Exp., expired. Mets., metastases. L, lymphocytes. P, plasma cells.
†Expired of uncertain cause. No autopsy performed.

TABLE 2. FOLLOW-UP IN PATIENTS WITH COLONIC CARCINOMA

	Without Metastases (Clinically Well)	With Metastases (Alive or Dead)
Less than 6 months	1	2
Less than 12 months	5	5
Less than 24 months	11	4
Less than 36 months	8	4
Total	25 (mean, 20 mos.)	15 (mean, 17 mos.)

B, and 21 as Dukes C. Seven were graded as Broders grade I, 31 as grade II, 5 as grade III, and 2 as grade IV. Twenty-four of the patients had preoperative CEA levels of 2.5 ng./ml. or greater.

In Figure 6 the cases are distributed according to Dukes classification and data plotted against the preoperative CEA values. Only one of the Dukes A patients had a CEA value above 2.5 ng./ml. and this case proved to be a Broders III tumor. Only 2 Dukes C patients had CEA levels below 2.5 ng./ml. and both cases proved to be Broders II tumors.

Figure 7 shows these cases classified by Broders grades of malignancy with

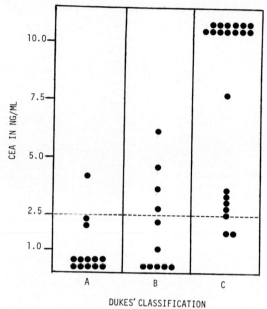

Fig. 6. Serum carcinoembryonic antigen (CEA) levels in 45 patients with colon cancer grouped according to Dukes' classification: *A*, growth limited to wall of colon; *B*, extension of growth through the muscularis propria but no metastases in regional lymph nodes; *C*, metastases in regional lymph nodes.

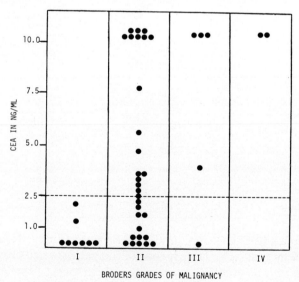

Fig. 7. Serum carcinoembryonic antigen (CEA) levels in 45 patients with colonic cancer separated into Broders' four grades of malignancy: grades I and II, well to moderately differentiated; grades III and IV, poorly differentiated.

the data plotted against the preoperative CEA values. All the 7 grade I patients had values below 2.5 ng./ml. and all were Dukes A. Of the 17 grade II patients with values above 2.5 ng./ml., 4 were Dukes B, and 13 were Dukes C. Of 4 grade III patients with values above 2.5ng./ml., 1 was a Dukes A and 3 were Dukes C. Both grade IV patients had values greater than 10 ng./ml. and were Dukes C.

Table 3 shows these cases correlated by CEA level and by Broders and Dukes classifications. All 7 Broders I cases were Dukes A, and the two Broders IV cases were Dukes C, with the intervening grades (Broders II and III) primarily Dukes B and C as expected. Characteristically most colon carcinomas are well differentiated; hence the majority of Dukes C cases were Broders II rather than III or IV. The CEA values correlated with both histologic parameters, but more with the depth of tumor penetration (Dukes). The CEA values were negative in all 12 patients with combined Dukes A and Broders I and II categories.

Figure 8 shows the direct relationship between CEA values and the presence of lymphatic, blood vessel, and perineural invasion. The 3 patients with no

TABLE 3. CORRELATION BETWEEN CEA LEVELS AND BRODERS AND DUKES CLASSIFICATIONS

| | Broders | | | | | | | | |
| | I CEA | | II CEA | | III CEA | | IV CEA | | |
Dukes	<2.5	>2.5	<2.5	>2.5	<2.5	>2.5	<2.5	>2.5	Total
A	7	0	5	0	0	1	0	0	13
B	0	0	6	4	1	0	0	0	11
C	0	0	2	14	0	3	0	2	21
Total	7	0	13	18	1	4	0	2	45

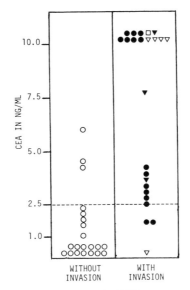

FIG. 8. Colon cancer: CEA levels versus lymphatic, blood vessel, and perineural invasion.

evidence of invasion and CEA values above 2.5 ng./ml. were Dukes-Broders A-III, B-II, and B-III.

Table 4 shows that invasion (lymphatic, blood vessel, or perineural) occurred in all 21 Dukes C tumors with none in any of the 13 Dukes A tumors. The correlation with Broders classification is less evident because of the large number of Dukes C cases in the Broders II group. None of the seven Broders I patients showed evidence of invasion, whereas invasion occurred in both Broders IV cases.

Table 5 presents the combined correlations of CEA levels, Dukes classification, tumor invasion (lymphatic, perineural, or blood vessel), and lymphocyte-plasma cell infiltration. Those tumors with invasion of the lymphatic vessels, blood vessels, or perineural space were predominately Dukes C and had minimal lymphocyte-plasma cell infiltration and high CEA values. Conversely, all tumors without invasion were Dukes A or B, largely CEA negative (18:3), and most had heavy lymphocyte-plasma cell infiltration (12:9).

The intensity of lymphocytic and plasma cell infiltration is compared with CEA values in Figure 9. Lymphocytes predominated with variable numbers of plasma cells present. No difference in the distribution of the two types of cells was apparent. The 2 patients with extensive lymphocyte-plasma cell infiltrates (2+ to 3+) and CEA values above 3 ng./ml. were Dukes C, and the one patient

TABLE 4. CORRELATIONS AMONG HISTOPATHOLOGIC PARAMETERS

		Dukes				Broders			
		A	B	C		I	II	III	IV
Invasion (L, V, or N)*	+	0	3	21	+	0	18	4	2
	−	13	8	0	−	7	13	1	0
		A	B	C		I	II	III	IV
Lymphocyte-plasma cell infiltration	(2+−3+)	8	4	3	(2+−3+)	7	7	1	0
	(0−1+)	5	7	18	(0−1+)	0	24	4	2

* L, lymphatic. V, blood vessel. N, perineural space.

TABLE 5. CORRELATION BETWEEN CEA LEVELS, DUKES CLASSIFICATION, TUMOR INVASION,* AND LYMPHOCYTE-PLASMA CELL INFILTRATION

	Dukes A		Dukes B		Dukes C			
	CEA <2.5	CEA >2.5	CEA <2.5	CEA >2.5	CEA <2.5	CEA >2.5	Total	Total
Invasion:								24
Infiltrate 2+−3	0	0	0	0	1	2	3	
Infiltrate 0−1+	0	0	1	2	1	17	21	
No invasion:								21
Infiltrate 2+−3+	8	0	4	0	0	0	12	
Infiltrate 0−1+	4	1	2	2	0	0	9	
Total	12	1	7	4	2	19		
Total	13		11		21			

*Lymphatic, vein, perineural space.

with CEA values greater than 10 ng./ml. was also Broders III with lymphatic invasion. Thus lymphocyte and plasma cell infiltration correlated directly with the degree of tumor differentiation (Broders), inversely with the extent of tumor invasion (Dukes), and inversely with preoperative serum CEA levels.

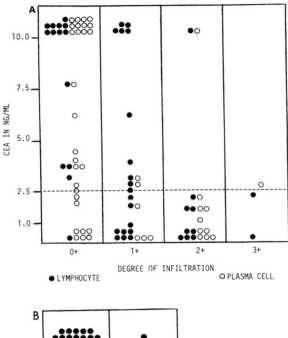

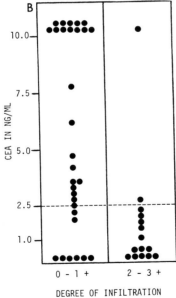

FIG. 9. Serum CEA levels in 45 patients with colonic cancer plotted according to the amount of lymphocyte and plasma cell infiltration on the advancing edges of the tumor, ranging from 0 (virtually no infiltrates) to 3+ (heavy infiltration). *A*, Lymphocytes and plasma cells graded independently. *B*, Combined grading of lymphocytes and plasma cells.

CLINICAL CORRELATES

Forty of the 45 patients were followed for 3 to 31 months (average, 17 months; Table 2). The other 5 patients were lost to follow-up and hence of uncertain tumor status. Of the 40 patients, 25 showed no clinical evidence of metastatic disease. Of the 15 patients who had evidence of metastases, 9 were alive and 6 were dead at the conclusion of the study. Table 6 shows the correlation between the immunohistopathologic studies of cancer of the colon and the clinical condition of the patients on follow-up.

The patients were divided into two groups: The 15 group A patients had known metastases. All the prognostic parameters in these patients were unfavorable: 85% were Dukes C, 93% had tumor invasion (blood vessel, lymphatics, perineural space), 80% had CEA levels greater than 2.5 ng./ml., and 93% showed minimal (0 to 1+) lymphocyte-plasma cell infiltration.

The 25 group B patients were clinically well and had no evidence of recurrent tumor. In these patients the prognostic parameters were favorable: 80% were Dukes A and B, 68% showed no tumor invasion (blood vessel, lymphatics, perineural space), 64% had CEA levels less than 2.5 ng./ml., and 52% had heavy (2+ to 3+) lymphocyte-plasma cell infiltration.

Table 7 presents an analysis of the prognostic parameters with regard to the depth of tumor invasion (Dukes), degree of differentiation (Broders), presence or absence of tissue invasion (lymphatic vessels, blood vessels, and perineural spaces), CEA levels, and lymphocyte-plasma cell infiltrate.

DISCUSSION

INTEGRATION OF PROGNOSTIC FACTORS

That gross and microscopic pathologic findings comprise the basis for clinical prognostication[10,35] is supported by our data. Preoperative CEA values also had prognostic significance. In addition, our data support the concept that tumor lymphocyte-plasma cell infiltration confers a favorable prognosis.[30] This study revealed that the pathologic evaluation correlated with CEA levels obtained prior to surgery and that the two sets of data together gave a better prognostic index than either alone. Patients with demonstrated metastases had higher frequencies of Dukes C tumor invasion, low levels of infiltration of round cells, and the highest CEA levels. Although the number of cases was small, the correlation was obvious and was supported by the available survival data.

TABLE 6. IMMUNOPATHOLOGY OF CANCER OF THE COLON: PROGNOSTIC CORRELATIONS

	Dukes Classification		Lymp. & Plasma Cell Infiltrate		Tumor Invasion		Preop. CEA Level (ng./ml.)		
	A&B	C	2±3+	0–1+	−	+	<2.5	2.5–5.0	>5.0
A. Known mets., 15 cases (alive or dead)		85% (13)		93% (14)		93% (14)		20% (3)	60% (9)
	15% (2)		7% (1)		7% (1)		20% (3)		
B. No known mets., 25 cases (clin. "well")		20% (5)		48% (12)		32% (8)		24% (6)	12% (3)
	80% (20)		52% (13)		68% (17)		64% (16)		

TABLE 7. ANALYSIS OF PROGNOSTIC PARAMETERS IN METASTATIC DISEASE

Parameter	% Patients Developing Metastases, Alive or Dead		Average Follow-up and Range in Months	
Dukes				
A	9	(1/11)	19	(5–31)
B	9	(1/11)	21	(9–28)
C	72	(13/18)	14	(4–28)
Broders				
I	17	(1/6)	17	(5–31)
II	36	(10/28)	17	(7–28)
III	50	(2/4)	19	(8–29)
IV	100	(2/2)	9	(4–14)
*Invasion of L, N, or V**				
None	5	(1/19)	19	(5–31)
L only	46	(6/13)	15	(8–25)
L + (V or N)	100	(5/5)	13	(3–27)
L + V + N	100	(3/3)	18	(12–28)
Lymphocyte and plasma cell infiltration				
L + P = 0	77	(10/13)	16	(3–28)
L + P = 1+ to 2+	31	(5/16)	20	(8–29)
L + P = 3+ to 4+	0	(0/11)	15	(5–31)
Preop. serum CEA (ng./ml.)				
<1	14	(2/14)	18	(5–28)
1 – 2.4	20	(1/5)	11	(7–22)
2.5 – 4.9	33	(3/9)	19	(9–29)
5 –10	50	(1/2)	24	(19–28)
>10	80	(8/10)	13	(3–25)

*Lymphatic, nerve, or vein.

CORRELATION OF CEA LEVEL AND DUKES CLASSIFICATION

Several reports have shown that when colonic tumors metastasize widely beyond the bowel wall, circulating CEA levels are elevated (2.5 ng./ml. or greater) in 83 to 100% of the cases.[8, 16, 19, 26, 36] The usefulness of the Dukes classification is well established, and the present series reaffirmed the correlation between the CEA level and the Dukes findings. In the present study, Dukes A and B cases were CEA positive in 7.6 and 36% of the instances, respectively, compared with 90% of the Dukes C cases.

CORRELATION OF CEA LEVEL AND BRODERS CLASSIFICATION

Broders' system for the histologic grading of tumor differentiation has been shown to correlate well with the prognosis, well differentiated tumors (I and II) being associated with longer survivals than poorly differentiated tumors (III and IV).[10] None of our 7 Broders I patients had CEA levels greater than 2.5 ng./ml. Two-thirds (30) of our cases were Broders II, and more than half of these (17) were CEA "positive." With one exception, our patients with poorly differentiated carcinoma (III and IV) had positive CEA tests.

In several previous studies of colonic carcinoma, no apparent relationship between the level of circulating CEA and the degree of tumor differentiation was reported.[8,16,19] In the present study we observed an inverse relation between the degree of differentiation and the circulating CEA level. This may in part be the result of differences in the methods of evaluation used. In our initial report the findings of "routine" pathology reports were used[8] In the present study, however, careful grading of the pathologic sections was done by more than one pathologist. The least differentiated tumors were not always associated with the highest circulating CEA values, since other factors also correlated with CEA levels, including depth of invasion, evidence of local lymph node and distant metastasis, lymphocyte-plasma cell infiltration, and other host factors. All must be considered in the prognostic appraisal of individual patients. Indeed, Martin and Martin[18] and Denk *et al*.[7] in a series of cases showed that the CEA content was lowest in their poorly differentiated tumors by both extraction and indirect immunofluorescence procedures. This apparent paradox requires further study. To account for our findings one must assume: (1.) that the total number of tumor metastases compensated for the small output of antigen of the anaplastic tumors, (2.) that these observations did not reflect the actual output of CEA by the tumor *in vivo,* or (3.) that other factors influence the circulating levels of CEA.

CORRELATION OF CEA LEVEL AND TUMOR INVASION

Grinnel,[12] Seefeld and Bargen,[27] and Sunderland[35] reported that the less the tumor differentiation, the more frequent the lymphatic, blood vessel, and perineural invasion. Our findings, similarly, showed that preoperative serum CEA levels tended to be higher when lymphatic, blood vessel, and perineural invasion was present. Indeed this observation implies that CEA values should be higher in less differentiated tumors (Broders III and IV), which are more likely to show local invasion. The obvious implication is that CEA gains access to the circulation via the common pathways of tumor spread.

CORRELATION OF CEA LEVEL AND LYMPHOCYTE-PLASMA CELL INFILTRATION

An inverse relationship was noted between preoperative CEA levels and the degree of lymphocyte and plasma cell infiltration in and around the subsequently resected tumors. This would seem to be paradoxical if one assumes that the round cell infiltrates reflect an immune response to tumor antigen. However, using the technique of lymphocyte transformation to study cell-mediated immunity to CEA, Lejtenyi *et al*.[15] found no significant response to CEA by lymphocytes taken from patients with gastrointestinal cancer, pregnant women, and normal individuals. Steward, Kupcik, Zamcheck[32] found similar results. Hollinshead *et al*.[14] observed skin reactions of the delayed hypersensitivity type in 17 of 19 patients with colonic carcinoma challenged intradermally with extracts from autologous tumors. Although positive skin tests were produced by several substances containing CEA, none occurred when "purified" CEA itself was used. The skin reactive antigen, which produced delayed hypersensitivity, was shown to be immunochemically different from CEA.[14, 24] Presumably then, the round cell infiltration reflects the local tissue responses to tumor constituents other than CEA. Alternately it may in fact be binding and destroying CEA, thus blocking CEA access to the circulation. The nature of the stimulus that triggers the cellular response to the malignant tumor is not yet known. Berg[2] has commented that "the closest the morphologist may come to seeing immunity is to see hyperplasia of some elements of the immune response."

PROGNOSTIC SIGNIFICANCE OF LYMPHOCYTE-PLASMA CELL INFILTRATION

A heavy round cell infiltration was prognostically useful; 13 of the 14 patients with extensive infiltrates were clinically well. Furthermore, 14 of the 15 patients with known metastases had little or no infiltrate. Fifty-two percent of the clinically "well" patients had 2+ and 3+ round cell infiltrates, whereas 48% had 0 to 1+ infiltrates. The infiltrate or its absence correlated predictably with both Dukes and Broders classifications, and the follow-up period was comparable in both groups. Longer follow-up is needed to determine whether the absence of a lymphocyte-plasma cell infiltrate will continue to indicate a poor prognosis.

Willis[38] noted that lymphocytes were frequently found at the spreading margins of carcinomas, occurred in greater numbers in association with slowly growing tumors, and were relatively scanty or absent in the presence of rapidly growing anaplastic lesions. He acknowledged that many workers considered this lymphocytic response a specific defense reaction against the tumor, but suggested that it may be due to preexisting or coexisting inflammation or to the liberation of degenerating products or metabolites from the tumor itself or from damaged elements in the invaded tissue.

Black and Speer[4] showed that patients with breast or gastric cancers associated with an increased round cell infiltrate had prolonged survivals. Several other tumors were shown to carry a better prognosis when round cell infiltrates were present.[1,6,17] Boyd[5] reported spontaneous regression of cancers of the colon and breast, microscopic sections of which showed marked round cell infiltration. Several authors have reported regression or even resolution of tumors following induced cell-mediated immune responses and have concluded that these were due to the round cell infiltrate.[21, 22, 31, 37, 41]

The lymphoid response is not seen in most cancers and when present, although offering a favorable prognosis, does not appear to be completely effective.[2, 3] The theoretical considerations have been discussed by several authors.[11, 13, 23, 34, 39] The prognostic usefulness of the lymphocyte infiltration requires further study.

Because preoperative CEA levels may assist the surgeon in planning his surgical approach and the extent of exploration (including examination of the liver and draining lymph nodes), we recommend that more than one CEA determination be done preoperatively when possible. Not only is greater reliability provided, but rising values have added significance. Similarly, serial postoperative CEA levels may help in the detection of recurrent disease. Studies from this laboratory and elsewhere have indicated the prognostic usefulness of serial follow-up CEA levels[29] and their potential help in monitoring chemotherapy.[28, 33]

SUMMARY

Preoperative serum CEA values showed prognostic usefulness and correlated with established histopathologic prognostic parameters. CEA levels provide an additional useful prognostic index of a complex immunopathologic process. The best prognostic appraisal of the individual patient can be achieved by a complete assessment of all participating factors.

ACKNOWLEDGEMENT

We wish to thank Dr. Herbert Kupchik under whose direction the CEA assays were performed.

REFERENCES

1. Berg, J.: Inflammation and prognosis in breast cancer; a search for host resistance. *Cancer 12:* 714–720, 1963.
2. Berg, J. W.: Morphological evidence for immune response to breast cancer; a historical review. *Cancer 28:* 1453–1456, 1971.
3. Black, M. M., and Speer, F. O.: Immunology of cancer. *Surg. Gynecol. Obstet. 109:* 105, 1959.
4. Black, M. M., and Speer, F. O.: Structural representation of tumor-host relationship in gastric carcinoma. *Surg. Gynecol. Obstet. 102:* 599, 1956.
5. Boyd, W.: Spontaneous Regression of Cancer. Springfield, Illinois, Charles C Thomas, 1966.
6. Dayan, A. D.: Spontaneous regression of cancer. *Lancet 2:* 1083, 1966.
7. Denk, H., Tappeiner, G., Eckerstorfer, R., and Holzner, J. H.: Carcinoembryonic antigen (CEA) in gastrointestinal and extragastrointestinal tumors and its relationship to tumor-cell differentiation. *Int. J. Cancer 10:* 262–272, 1972.
8. Dhar, P., Moore, T. L., Zamcheck, N., and Kupchik, H.: Carcinoembryonic antigen (CEA) in colon cancer; use in preoperative and postoperative diagnosis and prognosis. *J.A.M.A. 221:* 31–35, 1972.
9. Dukes, C. E.: The classification of cancer of the rectum. *J. Pathol. Bacteriol. 35:* 323–332, 1932.
10. Dukes, C. E.: Histological grading of rectal cancer. *Proc. R. Soc. Med. 30:* 371–376, 1937.
11. Good, R. A., and Finstad, J.: Essential relationship between the lymphoid system, immunity, and malignancy. *Natl. Cancer Inst. Monogr. 31:* 41–58, 1969.
12. Grinnell, R. S.: The grading and prognosis of carcinoma of the colon and rectum. *Ann. Surg. 109:* 500–533, 1939.
13. Hellstrom, K. E., and Hellstrom, E.: Cellular immunity against tumor antigens. *Adv. Cancer Res. 12:* 167–223, 1969.
14. Hollinshead, A., Glen, D., Gold, P., et al.: Skin-reactive soluble antigen from intestinal cancer cell membranes and relationship to CEA. *Lancet 1:* 1191–1195, 1970.
15. Lejtenyi, G. M., Freedman, S. O., and Gold, P.: Response of lymphocytes from patients with gastrointestinal cancer to the CEA of the human digestive system. *Cancer 28:* 115–120, 1971.
16. LoGerfo, P., Krupey, J., and Hansen, H. J.: Demonstration of an antigen common to several varieties of neoplasia; assay using zirconyl phosphate gel. *N. Engl. J. Med. 285:* 138–144, 1971.
17. Lukes, R. J., and Butler, J. J.: The pathology and nomenclature of Hodgkin's disease. *Cancer Res. 26:* 1063–1081, 1966.
18. Martin, F., and Martin, M. S.: Radioimmunoassay of carcinoembryonic antigen in extracts of human colon and stomach. *Int. J. Cancer 9:* 641–647, 1972.
19. Moore, T. L., Kupchik, H. Z., Marcon, N., and Zamcheck, N.: Carcinoembryonic antigen assay in cancer of colon and pancreas and other digestive tract disorders. *Am. J. Dig. Dis. 16:* 1–7, 1971.
20. Morson, B. C., and Dawson, I. M. P.: Gastrointestinal Pathology, pp. 558–564. Oxford, Blackwell Scientific Publications, 1972.
21. Morton, D. L.: Immunotherapy of cancer: present status and future potential. *Cancer 30:* 1647–1655, 1972.
22. Morton, D. L., Malmgren, R. A., et al.: Immunological factors which influence response to immunotherapy in malignant melanoma. *Surgery 68:* 158–164, 1970.
23. Piessens, W. F.: Evidence for human cancer immunity; a review. *Cancer 26:* 1212–1220, 1970.
24. Prehn, R.: Tumor-specific antigens and the homograft reaction. *Am. J. Surg. 105:* 184–191, 1963.

25. Rankin, F. W., and Broders, A. C.: Factors influencing prognosis in carcinoma of rectum. *Surg. Gynecol. Obstet 46:* 660, 1928.
26. Reynoso, G., Chu, T. M., Holyoke, D., et al.: Carcinoembryonic antigens in patients with different cancers. *J.A.M.A. 220:* 361–365, 1972.
27. Seefeld, P. H., and Bargen, J. A.: The spread of carcinoma of the rectum; invasion of lymphatics, veins and nerves. *Ann. Surg. 118:* 76–90, 1943.
28. Skarin, A. T., Delwiche, R., Zamcheck, N., Lokich, J. J., and Frei, E.: Carcinoembryonic antigen; clinical correlation with chemotherapy for metastatic gastrointestinal cancer. *Cancer 33:* 1239–1245, 1974.
29. Sorokin, J. J., Sugarbaker, P. H., Zamcheck, N., Pisick, M., Kupchik, H. Z., and Moore, F. D.: Use of serial CEA assays in the detection of recurrence following resection of colon cancer. *J.A.M.A. 228:* 49–53, 1974.
30. Spratt, J. S., and Spjut, H. J.: Prevalence and prognosis of individual clinical and pathological variables associated with colorectal carcinoma. *Cancer 20:* 1976–1985, 1967.
31. Sterjernsward, J., and Levin, A.: Delayed hypersensitivity-induced regression of human neoplasms. *Cancer 28:* 628–640, 1971.
32. Steward, A. M., Kupchik, H. Z., and Zamcheck, N.: Circulating carcinoembryonic antigen levels and serum suppression of phytohemagglutinin-stimulated lymphocyte DNA synthesis; an inverse correlation in the cancer patient. *J. Natl. Cancer Inst 53:* 3–9, 1974.
33. Steward, A. M., Nixon, D., Zamcheck, N., and Aisenberg, A.: Carcinoembryonic antigen in breast cancer patients; serum levels and disease progress. *Cancer 33:* 1246–1252, 1974.
34. Southam, C.: Relationship of immunology to cancer. *Cancer Res. 20:* 271–291, 1960.
35. Sunderland, D. A.: The significance of vein invasion by cancer of the rectum and sigmoid. *Cancer 2:* 429–437, 1949.
36. Thomson, D. M. P., Krupey, J., Freedman, S. O., et al.: The radioimmunoassay of circulating carcinoembryonic antigen of the human digestive system. *Proc. Natl. Acad. Sci. U.S.A. 64:* 161–167, 1969.
37. Williams, A. C., and Klein, E.: Experiences with local chemotherapy and immunotherapy in premalignant lesions. *Cancer 25:* 451–462, 1970.
38. Willis, R. A.: The Spread of Tumors in the Human Body. London, J. & A. Churchill Ltd., 1934.
39. Woodruff, M. F. A.: Immunological aspects of cancer. *Lancet 8:* 265–270, 1964.
40. Zamcheck, N., Moore, T. L., Dhar, P., and Kupchik, H.: Immunologic diagnosis and prognosis of human digestive tract cancer: carcinoembryonic antigen. *N. Engl. J. Med. 286:* 83–86, 1972.
41. Zbar, B., Bernstein, I. D., Bartlett, G. L., Hanna, M. G., and Rapp, H. J.: Immunotherapy of cancer; regression of intradermal tumors and prevention of growth of lymph node metastases after intralesional injection of living Mycobacterium bovis. *J. Natl Cancer Inst. 49:* 119–130, 1972.

ADDENDUM*

REFERENCES ON THE CLINICAL USE AND LIMITATIONS OF THE CEA ASSAY

1. Doos, W. G., Wolff, W. I., Shinya, H., DeChabon, A., Stenger, R. J., Gottlieb, L. S., and Zamcheck, N.: CEA levels in patients with colo-rectal polyps. *Cancer 36:* 1996–2003, 1976.
2. Herrera, M. A., Chu, T. M., and Holyoke, E. D.: Carcinoembryonic antigen (CEA) as a prognostic and monitoring test in clinically complete resection of colorectal carcinoma. *Ann. Surg. 183:* 5–9, 1976.
3. Mach, J. P., Jaeger, P. H., Bertholet, M. M., Ruegsegger, C. A., Looslie, R. M., and Pettavel, J.: Detection of recurrence of large bowel carcinoma by radioimmunoassay of circulating carcinoembryonic antigen (CEA). *Lancet 2:* 535–540, 1974.
4. Rieger, A., and Wahren, B.: CEA levels at recurrence and metastases; importance for detecting secondary disease. *Scand. J. Gastroenterol. 10:* 869–874, 1975.
5. Sorokin, J. J., Sugarbaker, P. H., Zamcheck, N., Pisick, M., Kupchik, H. Z., and Moore, F.

---

* A supplementary list of selected references is included as an Addendum for the reader who wishes a review of the clinical use and limitations of the CEA assay.

D.: Serial carcinoembryonic antigen assays; use in detection of cancer recurrence. *J.A.M.A.* *228:* 49–53, 1974.

6. Zamcheck, N.: Carcinoembryonic antigen; quantitative variations in circulating levels in benign and malignant digestive tract diseases. *Adv. Intern. Med. 19:* 413–433, 1974.

7. Zamcheck, N.: The present status of CEA in diagnosis, prognosis, and evaluation of therapy. *Cancer 36:* 2460–2468, 1975.

8. Zamcheck, N., and Kupchik, H. Z.: Summary of clinical use and limitations of the carcinoembryonic antigen assay and some methodological considerations. In *Manual of Clinical Immunology,* edited by Rose, N. R., and Friedman, H., pp. 753–764. Washington D.C., American Society of Microbiology, 1976.

Chapter 11

The Classification and Significance of Gastric Polyps*

SI-CHUN MING

It is well recognized that a polypoid lesion in the stomach may be the result of a variety of processes involving either the mucosa or the tissue underneath it. Such processes include hemorrhage, edema, inflammation, and neoplasia of various cell types. The true nature of a polypoid lesion can be ascertained only by histologic examination. When used as a pathologic entity, the term gastric polyp refers to a benign mucosal lesion composed primarily of epithelial elements. Only such epithelial polyps will be discussed.

Gastric polyps are not common. Their incidence is given in Table 1. In the general adult population studied either in a radiologic survey[43, 51] or at autopsy,[40] the incidence is about 0.4%. In clinical patients, only 3% of gastric tumors are polyps, whereas carcinomas comprise 88%.[31] On the other hand, gastric polyps are more common in persons examined in radiologic surveys. In one report,[51] the fluoroscopic examination of 5020 asymptomatic persons, in the age range of 45 to 84 years, revealed 10 tumors in the stomach, 8 polyps, 1 carcinoma, and 1 sarcoma. In another report,[43] 12 polyps, 20 carcinomas, and 3 infiltrating lesions were found in 10,000 photofluorographic surveys. Since almost one-half of the patients surveyed were less than 50 years of age,[51] and the average age of clinical patients was about 60 years,[2, 12] it may be assumed that there is a rapid increase of gastric carcinoma in the older age group, while the incidence of gastric polyp remains relatively stationary.

There are two significant aspects to gastric polyps: their cause of various clinical symptoms, and their potential for malignant transformation. As far as the clinical manifestations are concerned, gastric polyps have a low morbidity. In about one-half of the cases the polyp is either asymptomatic or only incidental to other gastric lesions such as chronic gastritis and cancer. These conditions are more likely to cause symptoms than the coexisting polyp. Polyp-related symptoms are obstruction, when a large polyp is present at either the inlet or the outlet of the stomach, and bleeding due to erosion of the surface of the polyp.

The malignant potential of gastric polyp is a much more significant problem

* Supported in part by United States Public Health Service Grant No. 12923 from the National Cancer Institute.

TABLE 1. INCIDENCE OF GASTRIC POLYP

Autopsy[40]	0.25–0.80%
Radiologic survey[43, 51]	0.12–0.40%
Among all gastric tumors	
Clinical cases[31]	3.1%
Radiologic survey[43, 51]	27.3–80.0%
Among benign gastric tumors	
Clinical cases[31]	41.0%
Radiologic survey[43, 51]	64.0–85.7%

than the clinical symptoms. This potential, which can be evaluated only by pathologic studies, is the main focus of discussion in this presentation.

REVIEW OF LITERATURE

It was Menetrier[29] who, in 1888, called attention to the relationship between gastric polyp and carcinoma. He described two forms of gastric polyps: polyadénomes polypeux and polyadénomes en nappe. Carcinomas occurred in both conditions. Polyadénomes en nappe, now recognized as Menetrier's disease, is a rare form of diffuse mucosal hyperplasia. Polyadénomes polypeux are discrete polyps. They are more common and their malignant potential has been the center of much discussion. There have been many reports supporting the view that gastric polyps are premalignant because of the presence of malignant change in them, ranging from 6 to 16%.[2, 12, 19, 21, 22, 26, 44, 53] Such a finding was not observed by others, however.[6, 37, 40] Some authors considered the presence of separate carcinoma in the same stomach also as evidence,[12, 22, 39,53] making the incidence of malignant transformation from gastric polyp as high as 51%.[39] On the other hand, it has been suggested that a stomach with a polyp may be more vulnerable to carcinogenic stimulation than one without a polyp[30, 45] and that the polyp is not the origin of carcinoma.[25, 45] The question of malignant transformation in polyp could have been resolved by histologic studies. Unfortunately, there has not been a uniform criterion. To some investigators, atypical epithelium and carcinoma in situ were evidences of malignancy:[2, 42] while others disputed their significance.[32] In most reports, the criterion for malignant change was not stated.

Since some gastric polyps become malignant and others do not, attempts have been made to distinguish between these two groups. Many of the early efforts were made without the benefit of histologic study, and attention was focused on two parameters: the size and number of polyps. It has been repeatedly pointed out that the larger polyps are more likely to have malignant change, and 2 cm. is often mentioned as a dividing point.[12, 16, 26, 32, 42, 55] Exceptions are common, however.[4, 16, 25, 26, 42, 44, 48, 59] Furthermore, polypoid lesions less than 2 cm. in size may actually be carcinomas.[27, 42] There have been discrepancies also among reports concerning the relationship between the number of polyps and their malignant potential. While most reports indicated a higher incidence of malignant change among cases with multiple polyps,[6, 12, 19, 26] others showed no such relationship.[2, 16, 55] Thus, neither the size nor the number of polyps are reliable indicators of their malignant potential. Furthermore, some polyps had been observed for as long as 23 years without either change in their appearance or development of carcinoma in them.[6, 12, 14, 32, 40]

It is apparent that for a long time there had been no reliable criteria to differentiate the polyps which remained benign from those which might become malignant. Since malignant change is a cellular event, the question of malignant potential must be evaluated histologically. Such an evaluation was presented by Rieniets and Broders[42] in 1945 and 1946. They divided gastric polyps into 18 different types which were grouped into two basic forms: one was simply called adenoma, composed of hyperplastic gastric glands and tubules, and the other was called papillary adenoma. Malignant transformation was common in the latter. The papillary lesions reported by others were reviewed by Walk in 1951 under the name of villous tumor.[59] They grew slowly and malignant changes were present in 60% of cases, irrespective of the patient's age. In 1959, Morson[34] divided gastric polyps into 2 types. For the first time an intestinal type of polyp was described. It was composed of intestinal glands, apparently having originated from the metaplastic epithelium. The other type was composed of true gastric epithelium. Carcinoma developed much more frequently in the intestinal type of polyp than in the gastric type. In 1960, Sagaidak[48] separated gastric polyps into 3 groups: adenoma, glandulo-fibrous polyp, and mucosal hyperplasia. Malignant change was present in the adenoma only. In 1965, Ming and Goldman[30] separated gastric polyps into 2 types: regenerative polyp and adenomatous polyp. For the first time, the neoplastic nature of the former, a common type of polyp, was questioned. This form of gastric polyp was recognized also by Nakamura[36] who called it Type 1 polyp. In addition, he described two other types: Type 2 polyp with a dimpled top, and Type 3 polyp with a flat or flower-bed gross appearance and marked cellular atypism. The Type 3 polyp was called atypical epithelium by Sugano, Nakamura, and Tokagi.[54] Tomasulo[55] also divided gastric polyps into 2 types: hyperplastic polyp and adenomatous polyp. The hyperplastic polyp corresponds to the regenerative polyp of Ming and Goldman.[30] From these studies it is clear that gastric polyps are not homogenous. They can be readily separated into 2 basic types, each with different cell composition, growth pattern, and malignant potential. Occasionally, both types of polyps may be present in the same stomach.[25, 30, 42, 55] Their different growth patterns are reflected by their gross appearance, making it possible to differentiate them without much difficulty radiologically and gastroscopically.[25] It is realized also that carcinoma develops frequently in the stomach away from the polyp, particularly when adenoma is present. The statistical data on these features are listed in Table 2.

In recent years, there is increasing awareness that gastric polyp may occur as a part of diffuse gastrointestinal polyposis,[5] either in hereditary syndromes or as nonhereditary conditions. The histologic appearance of most of these gastric polyps suggests that they are hamartomas. Although these cases are rare, it is important to identify them so that the systemic nature of the disease may be recognized.

CLASSIFICATION

In the past, the terms gastric polyp and adenoma were used synonymously, and the term polyposis was often applied to multiple polyps, as well as to diffuse hyperplasia of gastric mucosa. Such ill-defined usage of terms should be discouraged. Since gastric polyps are heterogeneous and different types of polyps may be present in the same stomach, the polyps should be evaluated individually. A proposed classification of gastric polyps is given in Table 3. Each type has a distinct histologic composition which appears to reflect its biologic nature.

The basic characteristics of gastric polyps are listed below, followed by a detailed discssion of the various types and their associated conditions.

Hyperplastic polyp: This polyp is composed of well differentiated foveolar mucous cells and scattered pyloric glands. The stroma shows varying degrees of inflammation and ingrowth of muscularis mucosa. Erosion of the surface is common. Malignant change is very rare. Grossly, the polyp is small and smooth-surfaced. It may be sessile or pedunculated. It remains stationary or grows very slightly.

Adenoma: The adenoma is composed of poorly differntiated cells, many of which show features of intestinal metaplasia. Stroma is scanty and inflammation is mild. Focal malignant change with stromal invasion is common. Grossly, the adenoma may be flat, papillary, or villous. It is either sessile or broad-based. It grows slowly.

Hamartomatous polyp: This polyp is composed of well differentiated cells normally present in the area. The predominant elements may be either glandular or stromal. Malignant change is either absent or very rare.

Retention polyp: This polyp is composed primarily of dilated, often cystic

TABLE 2. REPORTED INCIDENCES OF MALIGNANT CHANGE AND COEXISTING CARCINOMA IN HYPERPLASTIC POLYP AND ADENOMA OF STOMACH

References	Malignant change in polyp		Coexisting carcinoma	
	Adenoma	Hyperplastic polyp	Adenoma	Hyperplastic polyp
54	6% (4/71)[b, c]		47% (29/62)[a]	
36	18% (6/34)[a, c]	3% (3/95)[a]	29% (10/34)[a]	23% (22/95)[a]
55	21% (5/23)[a]	0% (0/74)[a]	59% (10/17)[a]	28% (21/74)[a]
60	21% (23/108)[b]		48% (52/108)[b]	
25	25% (2/8)[b]	0% (0/124)[a]		
30	40% (4/10)[b]	0% (0/76)[b]	30% (3/10)[a]	8% (3/39)[a]
59	60% (40/67)[b]			
42	73% (33/45)[b]	4% (4/96)[b]		
48	75% (40/53)[b]	0% (0/32)[b]		
Total	19% (11/57)[a]	1% (3/293)[a]	42% (52/123)[a]	22% (46/208)[a]
	41% (150/362)[b]	2% (4/204)[b]	48% (52/108)[b]	

[a] No. cases.
[b] No. polyps.
[c] Flat adenomas.

TABLE 3. CLASSIFICATION OF GASTRIC POLYP

1. Hyperplastic polyp
2. Adenoma
   A. Flat adenoma
   B. Papillary (villous) adenoma
3. Hamartomatous polyp
   A. Peutz-Jeghers polyp
   B. Juvenile polyp
4. Retention polyp
5. Heterotopic polyp

glands. The stroma is markedly edematous and may be inflamed. Malignant change is absent.

Heterotopic polyp: This polyp contains misplaced tissue from neighboring organs of the stomach. The heterotopic tissue may be located either in the mucosa or the submucosa. Malignant change is either absent or very rare. Since the component tissue is not gastric, it will not be discussed in this report.

HYPERPLASTIC POLYP

Hyperplastic polyp is the most common polyp seen in the stomach, comprising about 75 to 90% of gastric polyps.[25, 30, 36, 55]

HISTOLOGIC APPEARANCE

The hyperplastic polyp is covered on the surface with a single, smooth layer of surface epithelium and is composed primarily of markedly hyperplastic and elongated foveolar portions of gastric glands (Fig. 1). The cells are hypertrophied with abundant cytoplasm which is lightly eosinophilic and filled with

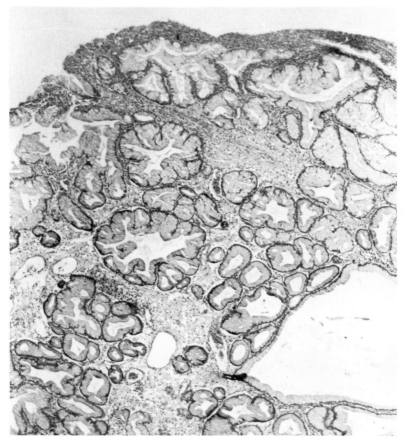

FIG. 1. Hyperplastic polyp. It is composed of hyperplastic foveolae, lined by a single layer of hypertrophic mucous cells. The cytoplasm is abundant and nuclei are small and basally located. Some foveolae show intraluminal infolding and cystic dilation. The edematous stroma is focally inflamed, especially under the surface. × 95.

neutral glycoprotein. The nuclei are small and basally located. Marked hyperplasia results in crowding of the cells which become narrow and tall but remain
in a single cell layer. In some areas the lining cells are cuboidal, the cytoplasm
contains fine eosinophilic granules, and the nuclei have prominent nucleoli.
They appear to be less differentiated mucous cells. Some foveolae are markedly
dilated and cystic. Intraluminal infolding and branching are frequently seen
(Fig. 2). In the deep portion of the polyp, small groups of pyloric glands are
common (Fig. 3) even if the polyp is located in the fundic mucosa. Serial sections
have revealed connections between the pyloric glands and some, but not all, of
the proliferating foveolae.[35] Chief cells and parietal cells are seen only rarely at
the base of a polyp located in the fundic mucosa. Mitotic figures are absent or
sparse. Intestinal metaplasia, occurring in about 20% of the polyps, is mild and
focal. The interstitum in the polyp is composed of loose connective tissue
infiltrated by chronic inflammatory cells, mainly lymphocytes, either scattered
or in aggregates. Occasional germinal centers may be present. The tip of the
polyp may be eroded with superficial necrosis and neutrophilic infiltration. In
such an area, immature cells with hyperchromatic nuclei and mitotic figures
may be present. Thin bundles of smooth muscle cells growing into the polyp
from the invaginated muscularis mucosa are often present (Fig. 4). The mucosa
surrounding the polyp shows a similar overall appearance to that of the polyp
itself in that there is mild hypertrophy and hyperplasia of foveolar cells, loss of
deep glands, focal mild intestinal metaplasia, and mild-to-moderate interstitial
inflammation. These changes merge imperceptibly with those in the polyp. The
absence of an abrupt change at the junction of the polyp and adjacent mucosa
makes it impossible to pinpoint the border of the polyp (Fig. 5).

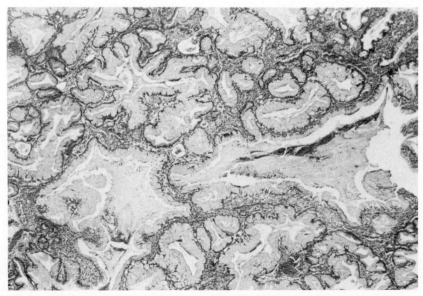

FIG. 2. Hyperplastic polyp. Branching and cystic dilation of foveoloae are present. The stroma is
infiltrated by many lymphocytes. Some foveolae also contain inflammatory cells. × 65.

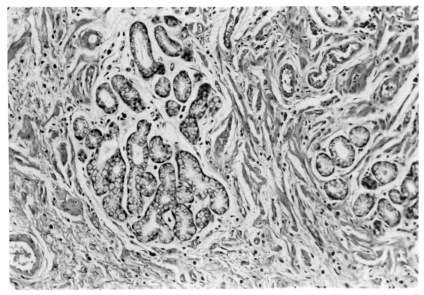

FIG. 3. Hyperplastic polyp. Groups of pyloric glands are separated by fibrous tissue and a few smooth muscle cells. × 260.

GROSS APPEARANCE

Gross appearance of the hyperplastic polyp may be predicated by its histologic appearance. The polyps are dome or olive-shaped with a smooth surface (Figs. 6 and 7). Their stationary nature is reflected by their small size, less than 1.5 cm. in diameter in over 90% of the cases. The small ones are usually sessile and the larger ones may be pedunculated. The dome of the polyp is sometimes red and depressed because of erosion, while the rest of the polyp is pink, similar to the surrounding mucosa, which may appear normal or atrophic. The hyperplastic polyp may be found anywhere in the stomach, but is slightly more common in the antrum.[44, 55] When it occurs in the fundic mucosa it often sits on a mucosal fold. In about two-thirds of the cases it is an isolated single lesion.[30, 36] In other cases, multiple polyps are present, usually less than 10.[32] It is rare to have numerous polyps, either confined to one area or diffusely scattered, in one stomach.

HISTOGENESIS

The histologic composition of hyperplastic polyps suggests that they are the result of excessive regeneration of foveolar cells following inflammatory destruction of gastric mucosa. This concept is supported by the following observations: (1.) Glands of similar histologic composition are commonly seen in the mucosa bordering a gastric ulcer or erosion,[35] and a hyperplastic polyp has been reported at the site of a healed ulcer.[33] (2.) The stroma commonly shows evidence of long-standing inflammation. (3.) Ingrowth of muscle cells from the muscularis mucosa is common. (4.) The polyp merges with the surrounding mucosa without a clear demarcating zone. (5.) The vast majority of polyps do not grow. (6.) The histologic appearance of the hyperplastic polyp is similar to that in Menetrier's

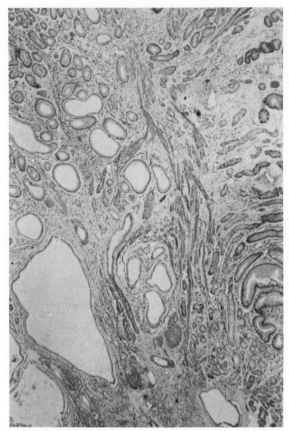

FIG. 4. Hyperplastic polyp. Irregular thin bundles of smooth muscle cells are present between hyperplastic foveolae, many of which are cystic. × 65.

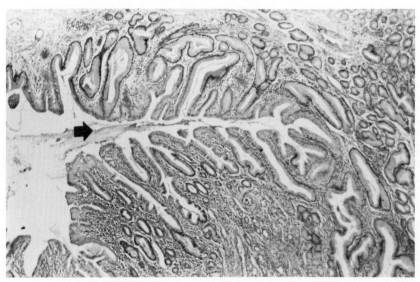

FIG. 5. Hyperplastic polyp. The deep groove (arrow) separates the base of the polyp above and the adjacent mucosa below. There is no difference between the two areas. × 65.

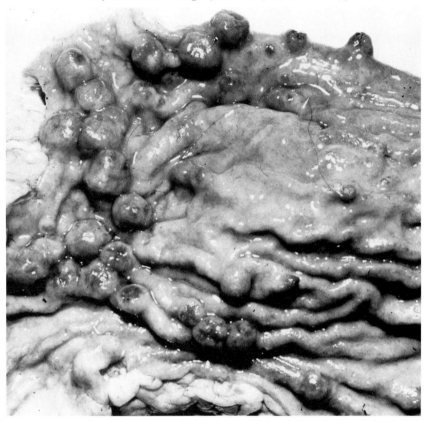

FIG. 6. Hyperplastic polyp. The stomach contains multiple sessile polyps, each has a diameter of 1 cm. or less. Some polyps are smooth-surfaced and others have erosion at top.

disease. All of these observations suggest that the hyperplastic polyp is not a true neoplasm. It is well known that the gastric mucosa heals and returns readily to its normal appearance. Why, then, in this situation is the repair excessive, resulting in the formation of a polyp? Alternatively, the hyperplastic polyp is a true neoplasm. In this case, one may wonder why it does not grow. To either question, the answer is not available. The persistence of inflammation in the polyp may have provided a continued but limited stimulation. In most cases there appears to be a balance between stimulus and growth, so that the polyp remains the same size for years. In any case, the hyperplastic polyp appears to be formed by circumferential expansion of mucosa due to uniform proliferation of many foveolae in one area. It enlarges slowly. When large, it becomes pedunculated and pulls muscularis mucosa into the stalk. The progressive stages of growth and the resultant gross forms are shown in Figure 8.

TYPES OF HYPERPLASTIC POLYP

Nakamura[36] has divided gastric polyps seen in Japan into 3 types. Type I polyp corresponds to the hyperplastic polyp described above. Type II polyp has a similar histologic appearance but there are a number of differences from Type I polyp. Type I polyps are mostly single, are situated in the antrum, and have a

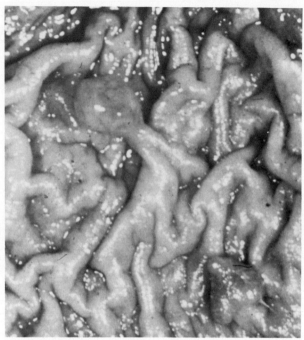

Fig. 7. Hyperplastic polyp. This stomach has two pedunculated polyps attached to the mucosal fold.

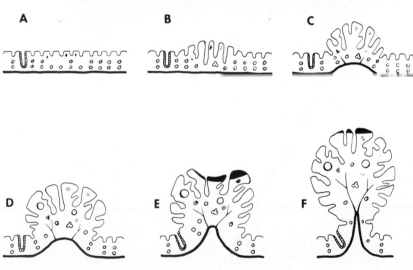

$\underline{\Upsilon}$ NORMAL GLAND, $\underline{\Upsilon}$ METAPLASTIC GLAND, — MUSCULARIS MUCOSA, ◼ ACUTE INFLAMMATION, ▨ CHRONIC INFLAMMATION.

Fig. 8. Hyperplastic polyp. Diagrams depict progression stages of development: A, original mucosa showing mild focal atrophy and intestinal metaplasia; B, mucosal hypertrophy with focal loss of deep glands; C, dome-shaped sessile polyp; D, oval sessile polyp; E, sessile polyp with eroded top; and F, pedunculated polyp. There is increasing foveolar hyperplasia with elongation, branching, and cystic dilatation. Residual pyloric glands are sometimes hyperplastic also. Inflammation in the stroma and ingrowth of muscularis mucosa are common. There is no demarcation between base of the polyp and adjacent mucosa.

smooth surface, whereas type II polyps are mostly multiple, are situated in the body of the stomach, and have a depressed erosion at the tip. The glands in the center of type II polyps have a concentric arrangement. Very likely, they merely represent variants of hyperplastic polyps, one with and the other without erosion at the tip of the polyp. Such erosions are common irrespective of the location or number of polyps. Type III polyp of Nakamura will be discussed under adenoma. Elster[13] has applied the term hyperplastic polyp to one showing hyperplasia of foveolae only and the term hyperplasiogenous polyp to one showing hyperplasia of deep glands and stromal elements as well. The difference between these two types lies in the degree but not the nature of the change.

MALIGNANT POTENTIAL

Since the hyperplastic polyp probably represents an exaggerated reparative and not a neoplastic process, it is not a premalignant lesion. In most reports, no malignant change in the polyps has been seen.[25, 30, 48, 55] However rare instances of such a change have been reported.[36, 42] It probably occurs in only 1 to 2% of polyps. One example is shown in Figure 9. This polyp contains many hyperplastic foveolae, in some of which there was malignant change with focal stromal invasion. None of the reported cases showed metastases. More important than malignant change in the polyp is the presence of independent carcinoma in the same stomach, which occurs frequently, in up to one-quarter of the cases.[36, 55] It therefore appears that the hyperplastic polyp has a much lower malignant potential than the intervening mucosa. This feature also suggests that hyperplastic polyp and carcinoma are not related. Furthermore, several follow-up studies have not revealed malignant transformation in the polyp.[14, 25, 30, 32]

ADENOMA

Adenoma of the stomach comprises about 10 to 25% of the cases of gastric polyp.[25, 36, 55]

HISTOLOGIC APPEARANCE

The adenoma is composed of glands lined with poorly differentiated cells of apparent neoplastic nature. They are pleomorphic columnar cells with large hyperchromatic nuclei and slightly basophilic cytoplasm in which mucus is either absent or scant (Fig. 10). Pseudostratification is common and mitotic figures are frequent. Goblet cells and striated borders are frequently seen (Fig. 11). Paneth and argentaffin cells may be present also.[36, 60] These cells end abruptly at their junction with the adjacent uninvolved mucosa (Fig. 12), often pushing aside the neighboring normal cells. Within the polyp, small islands of uninvolved, but usually metaplastic, mucosa are sometimes present. Abrupt change from adenomatous mucosa to the uninvolved mucosa also exists in these areas. At the base of the adenoma, occasional pyloric glands are present. Cystic glands are uncommon. In the early lesion the neoplastic cells are located mainly in the superficial region of the mucosa and the surface of the adenoma is relatively flat (Fig. 13). When the lesion grows further, papillary and villous patterns become increasingly prominent (Figs. 14 and 15). The stroma within the papillary and villous fronds is delicate and usually shows only mild inflammation or none. The muscularis mucosa is mostly intact. The adjacent mucosa

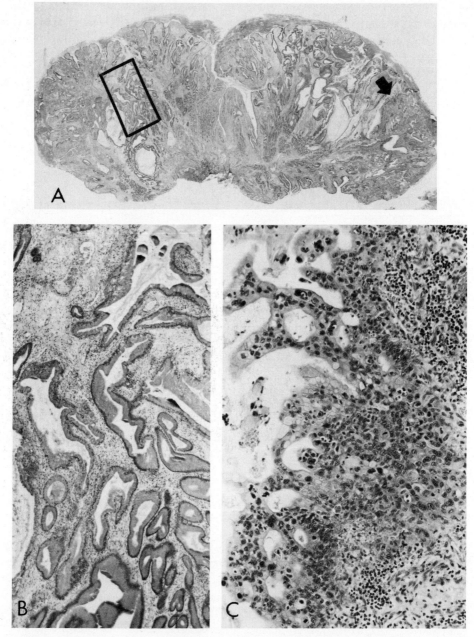

FIG. 9. Hyperplastic polyp with focal malignant change. This polyp measures 1.8 × 1.8 × 0.9 cm. Except for a deep fissure in the center, it has a smooth surface. Crowded glands and cystic areas are present. The left half is composed of hyperplastic foveolae typical of hyperplastic polyp. One representative area outlined in *A* is shown in *B*. In the right half many glands are lined with malignant cells with marked pleomorphism and many mitotic figures. In a few areas, stromal invasion is present. One such area, indicated by an arrow in *A* is shown in *C*. *A*, × 6, *B*, × 65, *C*, × 650. (Courtesy of Dr. I. Kline, Lankenau Hospital, Philadelphia, Pa.)

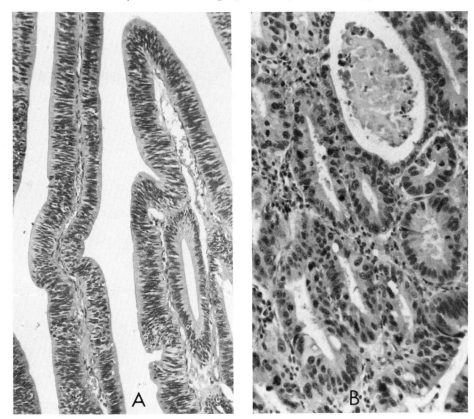

FIG. 10. Adenoma. *A*, cells covering the surface and lining the glands are poorly differentiated. There is marked pseudostratification. Cytoplasm is scanty and does not contain mucus. Villous formation is present. Stroma is scanty and not inflamed. × 260. *B*, The epithelial cells are immature. A few cells contain goblets of mucin. × 650.

generally shows chronic atrophic gastritis with prominent intestinal metaplasia (Fig. 16).

GROSS APPEARANCE

Adenomas are soft, velvety nodules, either sessile or broad based. The surface may be flat, papillary, or villous (Fig. 17). The crevices between the lumpy papillary projections often dip down to the base of the adenoma, corresponding to foci of uninvolved or slightly involved mucosa. In roentgenologic examination, radio-opaque meal is often trapped in these crevices, resulting in a soap bubble appearance to the lesion.[50] Watanabe[60] divided gastric adenomas into five groups: villous, pedunculated, flat, smooth sessile, and mammillated. Their respective incidences were 2, 7, 11, 17, and 63%. The flat adenomas are sessile, raised only slightly above the surrounding mucosa. Their surfaces are either smooth or irregular, resembling a flower bed.[36] They are relatively common in Japan, comprising over one-quarter of gastric polyps.[36] The majority are small, less than 2 cm. in diameter. Adenomas seen in other countries are often large,

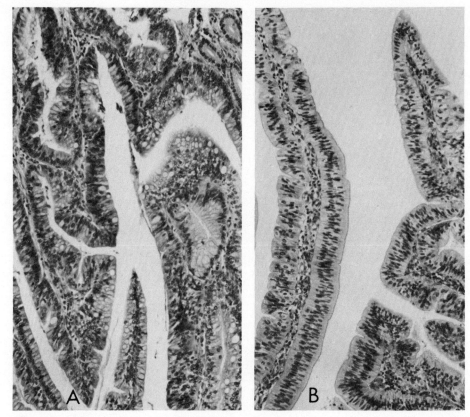

Fig. 11. Adenoma. *A*, many goblet cells are present. × 260. *B*, cells covering the villous projections show distinct striated border on the surface. × 260.

about one-half being larger than 4 cm.,[59] and adenomas as large as 15 cm. in greatest dimension have been reported.[28, 50] They occur as a single lesion in about two-thirds of the cases.[60] Most adenomas are located in the antrum.[55]

HISTOGENESIS

The resemblance between gastric and colonic adenomas is striking, particularly the papillary and villous patterns. The component cells in gastric adenoma are also of the intestinal type.[30, 34, 36, 56, 60] The surrounding mucosa, including residual mucosa within the adenoma, usually shows advanced atrophic gastritis and pronounced intestinal metaplasia.[30, 34] Thus, adenoma appears to originate from the metaplastic glands as first suggested by Morson.[34] The adenoma is a true neoplasm, since the cells are markedly dysplastic and proliferative and the tumor grows slowly.[59] The continued proliferative activity of adenoma is indicated by frequent mitotic figures. The appearance of adenoma cells pushing aside the normal cells at the transition zone indicates that they are able to grow along the basement membrane, replacing the surrounding cells. Thus adenoma is an expanding tumor, growing both vertically and horizontally. The growth rate has not been reported, however, since adenoma is generally resected on

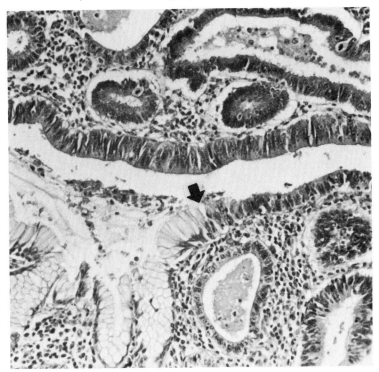

FIG. 12. Adenoma. The border of the adenoma (arrow) is clearly shown by an abrupt transition from immature adenoma cells to normal foveolar cells. × 380.

discovery. Local recurrence after resection, on the other hand, has been noted.[55, 59]

The presence of islands of uninvolved mucosa within the adenoma suggests that it is multicentric in origin. It probably begins at multiple points and by continued horizontal expansion the intervening mucosa is reduced to merely microscopic foci. The existence of such foci results in the formation of deep crevices and furrows characteristic of its gross appearance. The progressive stages of development are shown in Figure 18.

TYPES OF ADENOMA

Large adenomas are nodular, with papillary or villous projections on their surface; small ones are flat and only slightly elevated above the surrounding mucosa. The diversity of their gross appearance is probably determined by the duration of the lesion and the mode of expansion. When the lesion is early and small, it is seen as a flat adenoma, classified as Type III polyp by Nakamura,[36] manifesting primarily a horizontal growth. When vertical growth is pronounced, papillary or villous patterns become evident and the tumor may become pedunculated. Adenomas may therefore be divided into two major types: the flat type and the papillary or villous type. The primary importance of the division is chronologic. Both types may undergo malignant change, as will be discussed later. Lesions similar to flat adenomas have also been called atypical epithelium.[54]

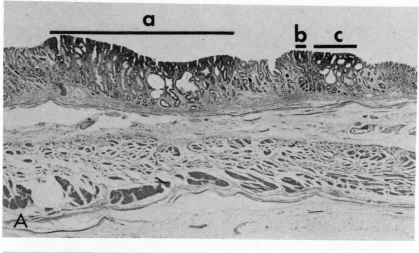

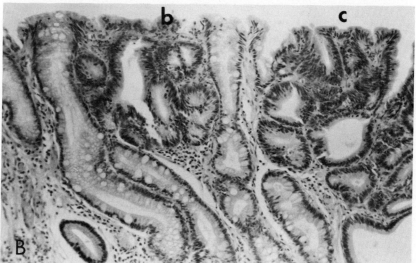

FIG. 13. Flat adenoma. *A*, three areas of adenoma are present in the atrophic mucosa. Area *b* and portion of area *c* are shown in *B*. The intervening mucosa shows marked intestinal metaplasia. The adenoma occupies upper one-third of mucosa. The lower portion of some glands is dilated. *A*, × 11, *B*, × 260. (Courtesy of Dr. K. Oota, Tokyo Metropolitan Institute of Gerontology, Japan).

MALIGNANT POTENTIAL

Adenoma is a true neoplasm. It is composed of immature and often abnormal cells and has the ability to grow and expand. Malignant change in adenoma is frequent (Fig. 19). The reported incidences range from 6 to 75%, with an average of 41% (Table 2). The lower incidences are seen in the small flat adenomas.[36, 54] Metastases are present in occasional cases. Of 10 cases studied by this author, 4 had carcinomatous areas, with extension into the submucosa in one and metastasis to a lymph node in another. Of 52 cases reviewed by Walk,[59] malignant change was reported in 40, and metastases in 5 cases.

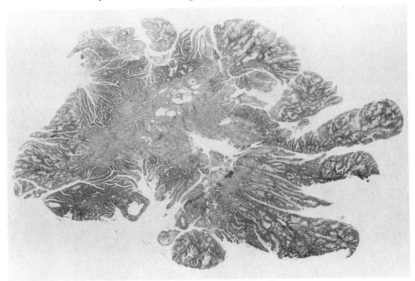

FIG. 14. Adenoma. The external surface is irregular, papillary in most areas, and villous in other areas. × 6.

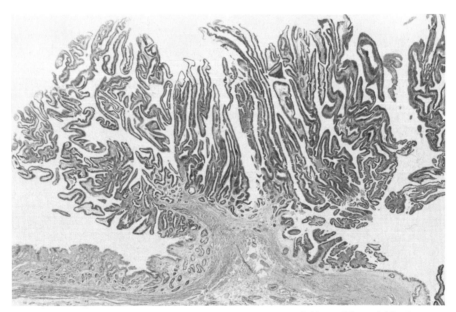

FIG. 15. Adenoma. Villous fronds are slender and stroma is delicate. The neighboring mucosa is atrophic, shown also in Figure 16. × 11.

The incidence of coexisting separate carcinoma in the same stomach is also high, occurring in 29 to 59% of cases (Table 2). This incidence is 2 to 3 times higher than that seen in stomachs containing hyperplastic polyps. The separate carcinoma may have originated in an adenoma, or alternatively, developed in a markedly atrophic and intestinalized mucosa which is particularly sensitive to

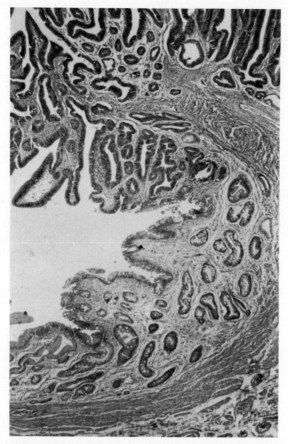

Fig. 16. Adenoma. Adenomatous tissue is shown in the upper half. The adjacent mucosa shows marked atrophy and intestinal metaplasia. × 95.

carcinogenic stimulation. Since both malignant change within adenoma and coexisting carcinoma are common, it is quite possible that both adenoma and carcinoma are induced by a common factor.

Gastric Polyp in Diffuse Gastrointestinal Polyposis

Patients with gastric polyp may have polyps in the intestine also. Among 50 cases of gastric polyp studied by Lawrence,[22] 9 patients had polyps in the intestine. Of 44 cases studied by Rieniets and Broaders[42] polyps of the small intestine, colon, or rectum were present in 23% and carcinomas in various parts of the gastrointestinal tract in 25%. In view of these observations, the latter authors suggested that the gastric polyp was only part of a general tendency for such patients to develop epithelial lesions. The nature of the intestinal polyps in these cases was not described and the genetic background was not evaluated. In recent years there have been several reports of cases with diffuse gastrointestinal polyposis.[5] Some of these conditions are hereditary while others are not. The gastric polyps in these cases fall into four types: hamartoma, juvenile polyp, retention polyp, and adenoma. In all of these conditions the polyps are multiple

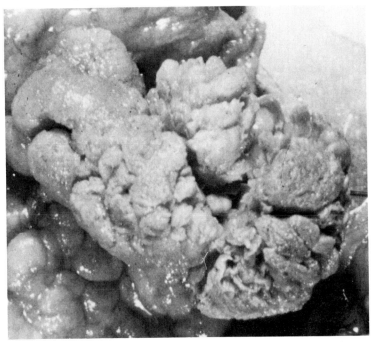

FIG. 17. Adenoma. It measures 4.5 × 2.7 × 2.0 cm. Deep fissures and furrows separate papillary lobules. Villous areas are also present. One such area is shown in Figure 15.

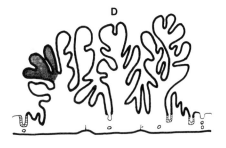

FIG. 18. Adenoma. Diagrams depict probable stages of development. *A*, adenoma probably originates from cells in surface epithelium and upper portion of metaplastic glands at multiple foci; *B*, flat adenoma is formed by horizontal spread of adenoma cells; *C*, villous adenoma is formed by vertical growth; and *D*, papillary adenoma is formed by either intramucosal growth of glands or expansion of villous fronds. Proliferation of muscularis mucosa is either absent or mild. Malignant change may occur at random areas.

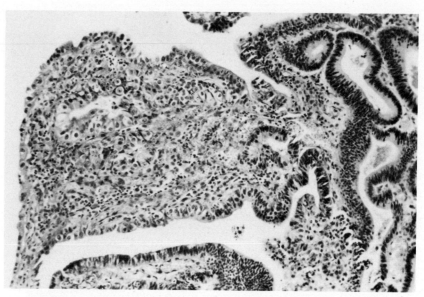

Fig. 19. Adenoma with malignant change. Malignant cells (at left) are mostly cuboidal or polygonal and have large pale nuclei whereas adenoma cells (at right and bottom) are columnar and have pseudostratified small nuclei. Stromal invasion by malignant cells is present. × 260.

TABLE 4. DIFFUSE GASTROINTESTINAL POLYPOSIS

I. Hereditary
　1. Peutz-Jeghers syndrome
　2. Juvenile polyposis
　　a. Childhood type
　　b. Infancy type
　3. Familial polyposis coli
　4. Gardner syndrome
II. Nonhereditary
　1. Cronkhite-Canada syndrome
　2. Random association

and their malignant potential is either uncertain or absent. The syndromes and conditions with diffuse gastrointestinal polyposis are listed in Table 4.

GASTRIC POLYP IN PEUTZ-JEGHERS SYNDROME

The polyps in Peutz-Jeghers syndrome are found mostly in the intestine.[20] They occur in the stomach in about 25% of cases. They are hamartomas, consisting mainly of densely packed glands normally present in the area.[5] Thus polyps in the fundic mucosa contain normal fundic glands and polyps in the pyloric mucosa contain pyloric glands (Fig. 20). The foveolar portion of the glands is often hyperplastic and focal atypism may be present rarely.[18] The glands are separated by irregular bundles of smooth muscle cells, extending from muscularis mucosa to the surface region of the polyp (Fig. 21). The muscularis mucosa at the base of the polyp and adjacent mucosa shows uneven thickness, and in some areas it is absent. Similar muscular irregularity is present also in the blood vessel walls. Fibrous tissue in the lamina propria is

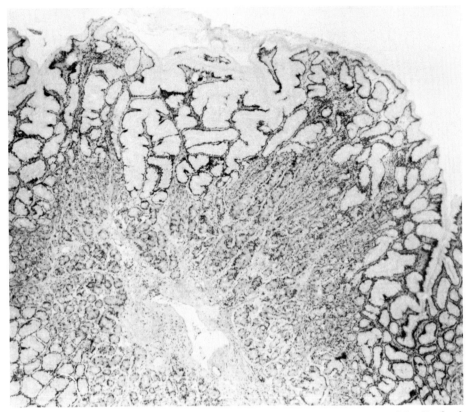

FIG. 20. Peutz-Jeghers polyp. This polyp in fundic mucosa is composed of normal fundic glands with hyperplastic foveolae. The stroma contains irregular vascular channels and thin bands of smooth muscle cells. × 65.

scant. Most polyps are small, less than 2 cm. in diameter. Their distribution is random. Occasionally, carcinoma develops in the gastrointestinal tract of these patients. Of 14 cases reviewed by Reid,[41] gastric carcinoma was present in 5 cases. In 3 cases the carcinoma had extended into the duodenum. The average age of patients with gastric carcinoma was 27 years,[20] and one patient was 13 years old,[1] which is much younger than patients with gastric carcinoma in the general population. Carcinoma of the colon or rectum occurred in only 2 cases in Reid's series.[41] Additonal cases of colonic carcinoma were reported by others.[10, 52, 57] Polyps of the colon in this syndrome have been reported as either hamartomas or adenomas,[10, 52] and it is possible that carcinoma may evolve from the adenoma. Adenoma has not been seen in the stomach, although the term adenomatous polyp has been used in earlier reports.[1] The relationship between gastric polyp and carcinoma in Peutz-Jeghers syndrome thus remains uncertain. If gastric carcinoma does not develop from a polyp, then these patients may have a general tendency to develop cancer due to other reasons. This possibility is supported by the finding of a high incidence of carcinoma in various organs in Japanese cases studied by Utsunomiya *et al.*;[57] 17 of 102 cases died with cancer, 1 in the stomach, 1 in the duodenum, 7 in the large bowel, and 8 in other organs.

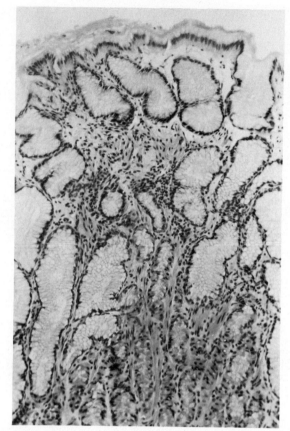

FIG. 21. Peutz-Jeghers polyp. Irregular bundles of smooth muscle cells between glands extend to the surface region. × 260.

GASTRIC POLYP IN JUVENILE POLYPOSIS OF THE GASTROINTESTINAL TRACT

Juvenile polyps are small hamartomas with prominent fibroblastic stroma, sparse cystic glands, and focal collections of lymphoid tissue.[35, 58] They often occur as isolated lesions in the colon of children. Multiple juvenile polyps may be present in members of the same family.[35] In such cases they may occur in the stomach and small intestine as well. The cases found in infancy appear to be autosomal dominant.[47, 63] The gastric polyps in these cases are multiple and small. Malignant changes have not been reported.

GASTRIC POLYP ASSOCIATED WITH FAMILIAL POLYPOSIS COLI

The colonic polyps in familial polyposis coli are adenomas. Recently, gastric polyps have been found in these cases. Boley *et al.*[3] reported 2 young siblings showing such a combination. Hoffman and Goligher[17] reported 3 young adults in whom gastric polyps were found 1 to 10 years after colectomy. Utsunomiya *et al.*[56] investigated the stomachs of 15 cases of familial polyposis coli in 6 Japanese families. Ten of these 15 cases were found to have multiple small gastric polyps, sometimes involving the entire stomach. Histologic examination revealed them to be flat adenomas. In patients with Gardner's syndrome, polyposis of the intestine is common and polyps in the stomach have been reported also, as either adenomas[61] or hamartomas.[38] Carcinoma of the stomach was not present in these cases, although it has been found in other members of the family.[15, 23] The malignant potential of gastric polyps associated with familial polyposis (adenomatosis) of the colon, therefore, is unknown.

GASTRIC POLYP IN CRONKHITE-CANADA SYNDROME

In Cronkhite-Canada syndrome there are multiple polyps in the gastrointestinal tract, particularly the colon, associated with ectodermal changes including pigmentation, alopecia, and onychotrophia.[8, 9, 20, 24] The gastric as well as the intestinal polyps are small, finger-like projections.[20] They are smooth-surfaced and edematous, resembling hydatidiform mole grossly.[24] Microscopically they are retention polyps, composed of dilated cystic glands and markedly edematous stroma. The syndrome occurs mainly in women during the sixth decade of life and is not hereditary. In one case, 3 carcinomas were present in the colon.[9] Gastric carcinoma has not been described.

HYPERPLASTIC GASTROPATHY

The gastric polyps described above are discrete circumscribed lesions. In hyperplastic gastropathy, the gastric mucosa is diffusely thickened. It is not a neoplastic condition. It is included in this discussion because the thickened gastric mucosa often takes on a polypoid appearance, sometimes erroneously interpreted as polyposis and because it may be complicated by carcinoma on rare occasions. The polypoid appearance of the gastric mucosa in this condition is mainly due to redundancy of mucosal folds.[11] It was described first by Menetrier who, impressed by the polypoid and ruffled appearance of the mucosa, gave it the name of polyadénomes en nappe.[29] It is now recognized that the same gross picture may be caused by 3 separate microscopic forms.[31] In one form there is a uniform increase of all cells, occurring as an asymptomatic, possibly congenital, condition. In the second form there is an increase of parietal and chief cells, but a normal complement of foveolar and surface cells. This form is seen in the Zollinger-Ellison syndrome. Hyperplasia of parietal cells appears to be due to increased gastrin stimulation. In the third form, there is an increase of mucous cells in foveolae which become enlarged and often cystic. A small number of pyloric glands are present. The broadened lamina propria shows inflammation and contains invaginated muscularis mucosae. These features resemble those seen in hyperplastic polyp. The last form was originally described by Menetrier and is now called Menetrier's disease. The chief clinical manifestation is loss of protein in the gastric secretion. The association of carcinoma with hyperplastic gastropathy was first reported by Menetrier.[29] Since then, additional cases have been reported.[7, 31, 46, 49] The histologic features of hyperplastic gastric mucosa in these cases have included all three forms. Such cases are rare and the relationship between carcinoma and hyperplastic mucosa is uncertain.

DISCUSSION

Gastric polyps are heterogeneous. There are at least four histologic types. It is important to separate them, since they have different clinical manifestations and malignant potential. Failure to distinguish them in the cases reported in the literature has made it difficult to analyze the data in these reports. Another difficulty is the lack of criteria for malignant change in the polyp. Cellular atypism has often been used as indicative of malignant change. It has been repeatedly said that such a change is limited to the tip of a polyp. If the polyp as a whole is premalignant, one would expect malignant transformation to occur randomly and not be limited to the tip. The immature or atypical cells at the tip of a polyp are probably regenerating cells occurring in an area of repeated trauma and erosion. They are not malignant. Such cells may be seen also at the edge of a healing ulcer. Although carcinoma cells are usually recognizable by their cytologic characteristics, it is not always easy to identify them with certainty. The best criterion for malignant change is invasion of these cells into the lamina propria or beyond. It has been cautioned that even local invasion does not indicate biologic malignancy, if metastasis is absent.[32] This interpretation is argumentative. Invasion is a biologic phenomenon. When it is limited within the polyp, metastasis is not to be exptected, a situation analogous to early superficial carcinoma of the stomach.

The most common gastric polyp is the hyperplastic polyp. The true nature of this polyp is not known. The high incidence of associated carcinoma in the same stomach may be cited as evidence supporting its neoplastic nature. On the other hand, the banal histologic appearance of the epithelium, the inflammatory stroma containing strands of smooth muscle cells, and the gradual transition of the polyp from the surrounding mucosa all strongly suggest the reparative rather than the neoplastic nature of this polyp. The term regenerative polyp was therefore applied to it.[30] Cancer develops in this type of polyp only rarely or not at all (Table 2). In fact, carcinoma occurs far more readily in the gastric mucosa away from the polyp than in the polyp. The reason for this phenomenon is not clear. There are two possibilities: one is that polyp and carcinoma are caused by the same factor and the other is that carcinoma develops separately in a susceptible mucosa. The latter is more likely because the gastric mucosa outside the polyp is often atrophic.[6, 42, 55, 62] A situation exists also for the development of gastric carcinoma in the absence of polyp. In any case, the stomach harboring a hyperplastic polyp should be carefully evaluated for separate malignant tumor.

The second most common gastric polyp is adenoma, a clearly neoplastic lesion. Gastric adenoma finds its complete analogue in the villous adenoma of the colon in that both are usually single, sessile and large, and both are prone to malignant transformation. Carcinoma develops randomly in the adenoma. Multiple sections of adenoma are often necessary to locate the malignant area. The cell composition of gastric adenoma strongly suggests that it develops in an area of intestinal metaplasia. Marked atrophy and intestinal metaplasia are common in the mucosa outside of the adenoma. Therefore it is not surprising that separate carcinoma occurs as frequently as carcinoma developing in adenoma.

In contrast to colonic carcinoma, adenoma is not a frequent precursor of gastric carcinoma. Nevertheless, it is no doubt one of the important causes. Of 17 cases of polypoid gastric carcinoma studied by Ming and Goldman,[30] 5 showed areas suggestive of residual adenoma (29%). A similar observation was made by Tomasulo.[55] Thus, perhaps one-fourth of polypoid carcinomas have their origin in adenomas.

The remaining two types of gastric polyp, hamartomatous and retention polyps, are rare. They occur in systemic syndromes involving not only the entire gastrointestinal tract, but other organs as well. They are not neoplastic and generally not premalignant. Although rare cases of gastrointestinal cancer have been reported in the Peutz-Jeghers syndrome, the relationship between hamartoma and carcinoma remains unclear.

CONCLUSION

Gastric polyps must be evaluated histologically if their significance is to be fully realized. Four types are described. Hyperplastic polyp is most common. Its malignant potential is minimal. Adenoma is a true neoplasm and frequently becomes malignant. Hamartoma and retention polyp are seen in diffuse gastrointestinal polyposis. Since the polyp often coexists with a carcinoma, the mucosa away from the polyp needs to be carefully examined also for the presence of a separate tumor.

REFERENCES

1. Achord, J. L., and Proctor, H. D.: Malignant degeneration and metastasis in Peutz-Jeghers syndrome. *Arch. Intern. Med. 111:* 498–502, 1963.
2. Berg, J. W.: Histologic aspects of the relation between gastric adenomatous polyps and gastric cancer. *Cancer 11:* 1149–1155, 1958.
3. Boley, S. J., McKinnon, W. M. P., and Marzulli, V. F.: The management of familial gastrointestinal polyposis involving stomach and colon. *Surgery 50:* 691–696, 1961.
4. Bowden, L: Adenocarcinoma in a small gastric polyp: A case report. *Cancer 15:* 468–471, 1962.
5. Bussey, H. J. R.: Gastrointestinal polyposis. *Gut 11:* 970–978, 1970.
6. Carey, J. B., and Hay, L.: Gastric polyps. *Gastroenterology 10:* 102–107, 1948.
7. Chusid, E. L., Hirsch, R. L., and Colcher, H.: Spectrum of hypertrophic gastropathy; giant rugal folds, polyposis, and carcinoma of the stomach – case report and review of the literature. *Arch. Intern. Med. 114:* 621–628, 1964.
8. Cronkhite, L. W., and Canada, W. J.: Generalized gastrointestinal polyposis; an unusual syndrome of polyposis, pigmentation, alopecia and onychotrophia. *N. Engl. J. Med. 252:* 1011–1015, 1955.
9. Da Cruz, G. M. G.: Generalized gastrointestinal polyposis; an unusual syndrome of adenomatous polyposis, alopecia and onychorotrophia. *Am. J. Gastroenterol. 47:* 504–510, 1967.
10. Dodds, W. J., Schulte, W. J., Hensley, G. T., and Hogan, W. J.: Peutz-Jeghers syndrome and gastrointestinal malignancy. *Am. J. Roentgenol. Radium Ther. Nucl. Med. 115:* 374–377, 1972.
11. Du Plessis, D. J., and Lawson, H. H.: Gastric mucosal alterations: benign and malignant. *Surg. Ann. 6:* 73–101, 1974.
12. Eklöf, O.: Benign tumours of the stomach and duodenum; a clinical and roentgenographic study with special reference to adenomatous polyps and the relation to malignancy. *Acta Chir. Scand. (Suppl.) 291:* 1–57, 1962.
13. Elster, K.: A new approach to the classification of gastric polyps. *Endoscopy 6:* 44–47, 1974.
14. Ferrucci, J. T. Jr.: Gastric polyps followed 20 years. *J.A.M.A. 199:* 207–209, 1967.
15. Gardner, E. J., and Richards, R. C.: Multiple cutaneous and subcutaneous lesions occurring simultaneously with hereditary polyposis and osteomatosis. *Am. J. Hum. Genet. 5:* 139–147, 1953.
16. Hay, L. J.: Polyps and adenomas of the stomach. *Surgery 33:* 446–467, 1953.
17. Hoffmann, D. C., and Goligher, J. C.: Polyposis of the stomach and small intestine in association with familial polyposis coli. *Br. J. Surg. 58:* 126–128, 1971.
18. Horn, R. C. Jr., Payne, W. A., and Fine, G.: The Peutz-Jeghers syndrome (gastrointestinal polyposis with mucocutaneous pigmentation); report of a case terminating with disseminated gastrointestinal cancer. *Arch. Pathol. 76:* 29–37, 1963.

19. Huppler, G. E., Priestley, J. T., Morlock, C. G., and Gage, R. P.: Diagnosis and results of treatment in gastric polyps. *Surg. Gynecol. Obstet. 110:* 309–313, 1960.
20. Jarnum, S., and Jensen, H.: Diffuse gastrointestinal polyposis with ectodermal changes; a case with severe malabsorption and enteric loss of plasma proteins and electrolytes. *Gastroenterology 50:* 107–118, 1966.
21. Kiefer, E. D., and Christiansen, P. A.: Benign tumors of the stomach and duodenum. *Med. Clin. North Am. 40:* 381–389, 1956.
22. Lawrence, J. C.: Gastrointestinal polyps; statistical study of malignancy incidence. *Am. J. Surg. 31:* 499–505, 1936.
23. Lindberg, B., and Kock, N. G.: A family with atypical colonic polyposis and gastric cancer; a three-decade followup. *Cancer 35:* 255–259, 1975.
24. Manousos, O., and Webster, C. U.: Diffuse gastrointestinal polyposis with ectodermal changes. *Gut 7:* 375–379, 1966.
25. Marshak, R. H., and Feldman, F.: Gastric polyps. *Am. J. Dig. Dis. 10:* 909–935, 1965.
26. McNeer, G., Joly, D. J., and Berg, J. W.: The significance of adenomatous polyps. In *Neoplasm of the Stomach,* Chapter 4, edited by McNeer, G., and Pack, G. T., pp. 56–68. Philadelphia, J. B. Lippincott Co., 1967.
27. McNeer, G., and Joly, D. J.: The problem posed by the small polypoid gastric tumor. In *Neoplasm of the Stomach,* Chapter 16, edited by McNeer, G., and Pack, G. T., pp. 238–243, Philadelphia, J. B. Lippincott Co., 1967.
28. Meltzer, A. D., Ostrum, B. J., and Isard, H. J.: Villous tumors of the stomach and duodenum; report of three cases. *Radiology 87:* 511–513, 1966.
29. Menetrier, P.: Des polyadénomas gastriques et de leurs rapports avec le cancer de l'estomac. *Arch. de Physiol. Norm. et Path. Par. 1:* 32–55 and 236–262, 1888.
30. Ming, S.-C., and Goldman, H.: Gastric polyps; A histogenetic classification and its relation to carcinoma. *Cancer 18:* 721–726, 1965.
31. Ming, S.-C.: Tumors of the esophagus and stomach. In *Atlas of Tumor Pathology,* 2nd series, Fascicle 7, pp. 81–154. Washington, D. C., Armed Forces Institute of Pathology, 1973.
32. Monaco, A. P., Roth, S. I., Castleman, and Welch, C. E.: Adenomatous polyps of the stomach; a clinical and pathological study of 153 cases *Cancer 15:* 456–467, 1962.
33. Mori, K., Shinya, H., and Wolff, W. I.: Polypoid reparative mucosal proliferation at the site of a healed gastric ulcer; sequential gastroscopic, radiological and histological observation. *Gastroenterology 61:* 523–529, 1971.
34. Morson, B. C.: Gastric polyps composed of intestinal epithelium. *Br. J. Cancer 9:* 550–557, 1955.
35. Muto, T. and Oota, K.: Polypogenesis of gastric mucosa. *Gann 61:* 435–442, 1970.
36. Nakamura, T.: Pathohistologische Einteilung der Magenpolypen mit spezifischer Betrachtung ihrer malignen Entartung. *Chirurg. 41:* 122–130, 1970.
37. Niemetz, D., and Wharton, G. K.: Benign gastric polyps. *Ann. Intern. Med. 42:* 339–344. 1955.
38. Parks, T. G., Bussey, H. J. R., and Lockhart-Mummery, H. E.: Familial polyposis coli associated with extracolonic abnormalities. *Gut 11:* 323–329, 1970.
39. Pearl, F. L., and Brunn, H.: Multiple gastric polyposis; a supplementary report of 41 cases, including 3 new personal cases. *Surg. Gynecol. Obstet. 76:* 257–281, 1943.
40. Plachta, A., and Speer, F. D.: Gastric polyps and their relationship to carcinoma of the stomach; review of literature and report of 65 cases. *Am. J. Gastroenterol. 28:* 160–175, 1957.
41. Reid, J. D.: Intestinal carcinoma in the Peutz-Jeghers syndrome. *J.A.M.A. 229:* 833–834, 1974.
42. Rieniets, J. H., and Broaders, A. C. Gastric adenomas: A pathologic study. *Western J. Surg. Obstet. and Gynecol. 53:* 163–170, 1945 and *54:* 21–39, 1946.
43. Roach. J. F., Sloan, R. D., Morgan, R. H.: The detection of gastric carcinoma by photofluorographic methods. III. Findings. *Am. J. Roentgenol. Radium Ther. Nucl. Med. 67:* 68–75, 1952.
44. Rosato, F. E., and Noto, J. A. Gastric polyps. *Am. J. Surg. 111:* 647–650, 1966.
45. Roxburgh, R. A.: The case for total gastrectomy in multiple polyposis of the stomach. *Gut 3:* 224–231, 1962.
46. Rubin, R. G., and Fink, H.: Giant hypertrophy of the gastric mucosa associated with carcinoma of the stomach. *Am. J. Gastroenterol. 47:* 379–388, 1967.
47. Sachatello, C. R., and Griffen, W. O. Jr.: Hereditary polypoid diseases of the gastrointestinal

tract; A working classification. *Am. J. Surg. 129:* 198–203, 1975.

48. Sagaidak, V. N.: Gastric polypi. *Probl. Oncol. 6:* 1155–1162, 1960.
49. Schindler, R.: Gastric carcinoma and gastritis: with reference to coexistence of carcinoma and chronic hypertrophic glandular gastritis. *Am. J. Dig. Dis. 10:* 607–624, 1965.
50. Shauffer, I. A., and O'Connor, S. J.: Villous tumor of the stomach. *Radiology 86:* 734–735, 1966.
51. Sherman, R. S., and Synder, R. E.: Roentgenologic surveys for gastric neoplasms; report of 31,895 examination. *J.A.M.A. 174:* 949–956, 1960.
52. Shibata, H. R., and Phillipa, M. J.: Peutz-Jeghers syndrome with jejunal and colonic adenocarcinomas. *Can. Med. Assoc. J. 103:* 285–287, 1970.
53. Stewart, M. J.: Observations on the relation of malignant disease to benign tumours of the intestinal tract. *Br. Med. J. 2:* 567–569, 1929.
54. Sugano, H., Nakamura, K., and Takagi, K.: An atypical epithelium of the stomach; a clinico-pathological entity. In *Gann Monograph on cancer Research: Early Gastric Cancer,* edited by Murakami, T., Vol. 11, pp. 257–269. Baltimore, University Park Press, 1971.
55. Tomasulo, J.: Gastric polyps; histologic types and their relationship to gastric carcinoma. *Cancer 27:* 1346–1355, 1971.
56. Utsunomiya, J., Maki, T., Iwama, T., Matsunaga, Y., Ichikawa, T., Shimomura, T., Hama-guchi, E., and Aoki, N.: Gastric lesion of familial polyposis coli. *Cancer 34:* 745–754, 1974.
57. Utsunomiya, J., Gocho, H, Miyanaga, T., Hamaguchi, E., Kashimure, A., Aoki, N., and Komatsu, I.: Peutz-Jeghers syndrome; its natural course and management. *Johns Hopkins Med. J. 136:* 71–82, 1975.
58. Veale, A. M. O., McColl, I., Bussey, H. J. R., and Morson, B. C.: Juvenile polyposis coli. *J. Med. Genet. 3:* 5–16, 1966.
59. Walk, L.: Villous tumor of the stomach. Clinical review and report of two cases. *Arch. Intern. Med. 87:* 560–569, 1951.
60. Watanabe, H.: Argentaffin cells in adenoma of the stomach. *Cancer 30:* 1267–1274, 1972.
61. Yaffee, H. S.: Gastric polyposis and soft tissue tumors; a variant of Gardner's syndrome. *Arch. Dermatol. 89:* 806–808, 1964.
62. Yarnis, H., Marshak, R. H., and Friedman, A. I.: Gastric polyps. *J.A.M.A. 148:* 1088–1094, 1952.
63. Yonemoto, R. H., Slayback, J. B., Byron, R. L. Jr., and Rosen, R. B.: Familial polyposis of the entire gastrointestinal tract. *Arch. Surg. 99:* 427–434, 1969.

Chapter 12

The Japanese Classification of Early Gastric Cancer

B. C. MORSON

Early gastric cancer is defined as a carcinoma which is confined to the mucosa, or mucosa and submucosa, regardless of the presence of lymphnode metastasis.[11] It must be emphasized that this is a classification of the gross or macroscopic appearance. Early gastric carcinoma can also be subdivided by microscopic criteria into two groups, intramucosal carcinoma and submucosal carcinoma, both with potential for lymphnode metastasis. It is now doubtful whether, for the stomach, the expression "carcinoma-in-situ" can ever be used with confidence because it is difficult and often impossible to be sure whether neoplastic cells have passed across the basement membrane of the crypts into the lamina propria of the mucous membrane. Invasion of the latter only, without extension into the submucosal layer, is commonly observed by Japanese pathologists with their great experience with early gastric cancer.

Surface carcinoma and superficial carcinoma are terms which have been used synonymously with intramucosal carcinoma. The expression *superficial spreading carcinoma* was introduced by Stout in 1942[19] to describe the type of carcinoma which spreads superficially in the mucosa and submucosa without penetrating the deep muscle layers until it has covered a considerable surface area. It could be regarded as an early manifestation of linitis plastica. It has little relevance to the Japanese classification.

It is important to get international agreement on the nomenclature and classification of tumors and my own experience, coupled with the study of the Japanese and European work on early gastric cancer, has led me to the view that the Japanese classification and nomenclature should be adopted as a worldwide practice. The reasons for this follow.

METHODS OF INVESTIGATION

The importance of careful examination of gastrectomy specimens cannot be overstressed otherwise early gastric cancer will be missed. Gastrectomy specimens should always be obtained fresh from the operating room and carefully cut along the greater curvature and pinned out on a cork board with the mucosal surface uppermost. Before and after fixation examination of the mucous membrane should be made for the slightest irregularities or surface erosion. A hand lens is useful for this purpose. It is essential to take up to 15 or 20 blocks of tissue, particularly from the lesser curve aspect and antral region of the stomach, and the origin of these must be mapped on an outline chart of the gastrectomy specimen. The Swiss roll technique[7] can be useful.

The frequency with which early gastric cancer is found depends in the first place on the interest shown by gastroenterologists, surgeons, and endoscopists. The pathologist can play his part by careful examination of gastrectomy specimens. The high incidence of gastric cancer in Japan and the enthusiasm there for gastroscopy has led to a situation in which about 30% of gastrectomies for carcinoma are for early disease. In Europe and North America the rate is certainly much less than 10%, even in specialist gastroenterology centers.

THE CLASSIFICATION OF EARLY GASTRIC CANCER

This classification was agreed to at a meeting of the Japan Gastroenterological Endoscopic Society in 1962.[11] Early gastric cancer was divided into three main groups and three subgroups on the basis of the macroscopic appearances at endoscopy and in gastrectomy specimens (Fig. 1).

TYPE I: THE PROTRUDED TYPE

The tumor projects clearly into the lumen. All polypoid, nodular, and villous tumors are included in this group. Perhaps the best nomenclature for the English literature would be protuberant or polypoid rather than protruded.

TYPE II: THE SUPERFICIAL TYPE

This is further subdivided into three subgroups:

Type II(a) Elevated. In carefully prepared gastrectomy specimens this is seen as a flat, plaque-like lesion, well circumscribed, and only raised above the surrounding mucosa by a few millimeters.

Type II(B) Flat. No abnormality is macroscopically visible, although some color change may be visible endoscopically and in very carefully prepared gastrectomy specimens.

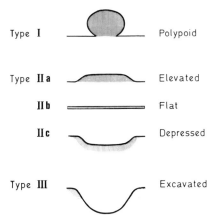

Type I		Polypoid
Type II a		Elevated
II b		Flat
II c		Depressed
Type III		Excavated

FIG. 1. Macroscopic classification of early gastric carcinoma.

Type II(C) Depressed. The surface is slightly depressed below the adjacent mucosa for not more than the thickness of the submucosa. Surface erosion may be apparent from a thin covering of exudate.

Type III: The Excavated Type

It is essentially ulceration of variable depth into the gastric wall. This is rarely seen in pure form and is almost always combined with any of the other types.

The Japanese invariably use the symbols of the classification and this becomes complex when a lesion has features of more than one type. Some combinations of types are commoner than a single type, and all possible combinations of the five types have been described. The dominant macroscopic feature is placed first. Thus, early gastric cancer can be described as I + IIc, or IIc + III, or IIa + IIc, etc. Combinations of three types are also seen.

For many pathologists this classification using numerals and alphabetical letters as symbols in various combinations has seemed complex to the point of being indigestible. Perhaps it is better that they should look at the classification in Figure 1 and use the descriptive terms rather than the symbols, but the latter are essential for the description of combinations of types.

This Japanese classification, and its modifications introduced by European authors, is now being widely adopted and it is essential that pathologists should understand and become familiar with it. This is necessary not only for reporting purposes, but also because the classification has relevance for the histogenesis of carcinoma of the stomach. The endoscopist and radiologist as well as the surgeon and gastroenterologist especially concerned with the diagnosis and treatment of gastric cancer require this sophisticated service from the pathologist.

It is important to remember that the type III early gastric carcinoma refers to the ulceration or excavation and not to the state of the surrounding mucosa. Thus, type III carcinomas should seldom be used alone, but in combination with another type, *e.g.,* III + IIc.

The classification of early gastric cancer can be used for lesions of any size, although most of them are about 2.0 cm. in diameter or less. Larger areas of up to 5 cm. in diameter are not uncommon. Most early gastric cancer will be found in the antrum and along the lesser curvature of the stomach and this is why it is so important that pathologists should be particularly alert for macroscopic abnormalities in these areas. About 10% of gastrectomy specimens for early gastric cancer will show multifocal lesions.

The relative frequency of the different macroscopic types of early gastric cancer varies with different authors and with different countries. The protuberant (type I) carcinomas account for between 10% and 15%, but the incidence given by European authors, Elster *et al.*[2] and Johansen,[4] is rather higher than that given by the Japanese.[13] Superficial (type II) carcinoma is commoner than type I but these are mostly type IIc (superficial, depressed) and slightly elevated and flat varieties of type II are relatively much less common. However, European authors report a much higher incidence of all superficial type early gastric cancers than do their Japanese colleagues. It has already been pointed out that type III early gastric cancer in its pure form is rare but all combinations with the other types are common. Thus, the combination forms, not unexpectedly, account for about 70% of all early gastric cancers in Japan and between 40% and 50% in the main European publications.[2, 4, 13] The excavating type of early gastric cancer is more commonly seen in Japan than in Europe, although usually in combination with other types. This should not be taken to mean that all excavating lesions are ulcer-cancers in the sense that the carcinoma arose from previously benign peptic ulcers. There is considerable disagreement among Japanese authors about the frequency of ulcer-cancer in Japan but if the strict criteria introduced by Newcomb[18] are observed the incidence is low.[16] This low incidence would conform with the current opinion of North American and European pathologists.

The relative incidence of the various types and combinations of types of early gastric carcinoma in different geographic areas could have epidemiologic importance and this is one reason why the Japanese classification should be adopted as a worldwide practice.

HISTOLOGY OF EARLY GASTRIC CANCER

Types I (protuberant) and IIa (superficial, elevated) early gastric carcinomas are almost invariably well differentiated adenocarcinomas. Among the type IIc (superficial, depressed), well differentiated, poorly differentiated, signet ring cell, and undifferentiated carcinomas are all seen, but the degree of differentiation in any one lesion is often variable.[2] The relative frequency of poorly differentiated and undifferentiated carcinomas is much higher among the type III (excavated) early gastric cancers than any of the other types in the classification. In general then, elevated carcinomas are usually well differentiated, depressed ones contain all histologic types, and excavating cancers have the highest incidence of poorly differentiated and undifferentiated carcinomas.

It must be emphasized that the gastric mucosa has to be very carefully scrutinized for evidence of intramucosal carcinoma, especially in the case of type II early gastric cancers. Invasion of the lamina propria only by undifferentiated or signet ring carcinoma cells in particular can be missed very easily. For this reason multiple sections of the mucosa around gastric ulcers should be examined for signs of intramucosal carcinoma. Similarly very careful scrutiny of gastric biopsies is essential and mucin stains can be helpful in the detection of isolated clumps of undifferentiated carcinoma cells in the lamina propria.

It is appropriate here to return to the problem of differentiating between epithelial atypia in gastric mucosa, carcinoma-in-situ, intramucosal carcinoma, and what many pathologists would call an adenoma of the stomach.

Epithelial atypia (dysplasia) is a useful term for the cellular changes which fall short of the full criteria for the diagnosis of carcinoma-in-situ. The latter must exist at some state in the progression of epithelial dysplasia of gastric mucosa into invasive carcinoma but, as already stated at the beginning of this chapter, it is usually impossible to be certain that the neoplastic cells have not passed across the basement membrane of the crypts into the lamina propria without serial sectioning of the entire lesion, which is impracticable. Probably this phase of carcinoma-in-situ in the stomach is an extremely short one.

For the reasons given it is recommended that the expression carcinoma-in-situ be dropped in favor of intramucosal carcinoma, provided that it is used only when lamina propria invasion has been demonstrated. For doubtful cases it is essential to examine multiple sections through the tissue. Even then, invasion may not be demonstrated and the pathologist is in a dilemma. The Japanese have recognized this problem and have introduced the expression "borderline lesion". For the purist that is an unsuitable expression for the description of a histologic appearance, but it does illustrate the problem. My study of the Japanese literature suggests that what the Japanese are describing might be called an adenoma by many European and North American pathologists. Although polypoid adenomas of the stomach do occur they are rare compared with their counterparts in the colon. They are usually tubulovillous or villoglandular in their histologic structure. The border line lesion of the Japanese pathologists appears to me to be more like a slightly elevated or even flat adenoma and would correspond to a type IIa or IIb early gastric cancer. It could be called intramu-cosal adenoma in order to distinguish it from polypoid adenoma. The macro-scopic or endoscopic classification thus has some relevance to the problems of classification of gastric polyps, especially the neoplastic group or adenomas. Our Japanese colleagues are currently observing the borderline lesion by regular gastric biopsy to see how it behaves and there is some evidence that it progresses to invasive carcinoma only slowly and in some cases possibly not at all, rather like the adenoma-carcinoma sequence in the large intestine.[11, 12]

THE IMPORTANCE OF THE JAPANESE CLASSIFICATION OF EARLY GASTRIC CANCER

FOR THE RADIOLOGIST

The double contrast technique of barium meal examination of the stomach can demonstrate small lesions so clearly that they resemble photographs of surgical specimens.[11] It is unfortunate that this method has not been more widely adopted by radiologists in Europe and the United States. Its wider use would undoubtedly increase the yield of early gastric carcinomas, which is lamentably low outside Japan.

FOR THE ENDOSCOPIST

Technical advances in the use of the fiberoptic gastroscope and its attach-ments have made it possible to observe the entire lining of the stomach with great precision. It is possible to take endoscopic photographs of high quality to illustrate the classification of early gastric cancer and this is a point of great interest for pathologists. Moreover, it is now possible to take biopsies from any part of the gastric mucosa under direct vision. Modern biopsy forceps can remove small pieces of tissue which are large enough to be correctly orientated and then embedded in wax in such a way that the histopathologist can observe the tissue in its normal microanatomic relationships. The method is essentially the same as that described for small bowel and rectal biopsies.[9]

FOR THE PATHOLOGIST

Close collaboration with the radiologist and endoscopist can give the patholo-gist reason to believe that a particular gastric biopsy may show the changes of early gastric cancer, particularly intramucosal carcinoma. This will, at least, alert him to the importance of obtaining the gastrectomy specimen fresh and preparing it carefully for examination and photography as already described. All biopsies should be carefully screened for evidence of malignant cells invading the lamina propria as these may be present in small numbers. However, the diagnosis of intramucosal carcinoma on a gastric biopsy is purely descriptive of what has been seen in the sample of tissue submitted and of course cannot be used to classify the patient as having early or advanced cancer of the stomach.

The cytologist has an important role to play in the diagnosis of early gastric cancer. The brush cytology technique probably gives the best results, but lavage and smear cytology are also very good methods. There should be no controversy about the relative merits of cytology and biopsy because these methods are complementary. Anyway, the choice and the success rate depends on the availability of expertise.

It is obvious that increased availability of intramucosal and other early gastric carcinomas should improve our knowledge of the histogenesis of carcinoma of the stomach. So far, however, research in recent years by Japanese and German workers in particular has not made any great advance on what is already known.

The concept that most gastric cancers arise on a basis of intestinal metaplasia was firmly established by Järvi and Laurén,[3] Morson,[8] and Elster *et al.*[1] Nakamura[14, 15, 17] with his much greater experience with early gastric carcinoma has confirmed this concept and emphasized that the better differentiated adenocarcinomas arise against a background of intestinal metaplasia whereas the poorly differentiated and undifferentiated tumors arise from ordinary gastric epithelium. This is almost certainly an oversimplification.

Laurén[6] subdivided carcinomas of the stomach into the intestinal type (53%) and the diffuse type (33%), with the remainder (14%) left out of the classification. In my experience, this histologic classification is difficult to apply accurately because of the great variability in the microscopic features of individual gastric cancers, but it does seem to have considerable epidemiologic importance. In countries with a high incidence of gastric cancer the intestinal type is very common, whereas the diffuse type is more prevalent in low risk areas.[10]

Although many gastric cancers arise from metaplastic intestinal epithelium it seems inherently unlikely that all of them do so, if only because intestinal metaplasia of the gastric mucosa is not found in all cases of cancer of the stomach. The study of early gastric carcinoma should provide information about alternative mechanisms of histogenesis from foveolar epithelium and undifferentiated cells at the base of the gastric crypts. It is possible that the mucus-secreting pyloric glands and even the specialized epithelial cells of the body mucosa could be the source of malignant tumors. Study of early gastric cancers by the light microscope, histochemical methods, and the electron microscope is required in order to further clarify the role of both metaplastic intestinal epithelium and ordinary gastric epithelial cells in the genesis of cancer of the stomach. Personally, I have no doubt that carcinoma of the stomach can arise from ordinary gastric epithelium, but the sequence of events is yet to be described.

POTENTIAL FOR LYMPHNODE METASTASIS

The incidence of lymphnode metastasis in early carcinoma varies with the depth of penetration into the wall of the stomach. In cases of intramucosal carcinoma lymphnode involvement is exceptional but can occur. Kidokoro[5] reported only 1 example in 32 cases. In contrast, the same author found a 12% incidence of metastasis to regional lymphnodes in a large series of submucosal cancers collected from 22 hospitals. Advanced gastric cancers have a very high frequency of lymphnode involvement of the order of 60 to 70%.

PROGNOSIS AFTER SURGICAL TREATMENT

The 5-year survival rate after surgical treatment for early gastric carcinoma is about 95%.[5] Recurrence after treatment for intramucosal carcinoma is very rare and most of the deaths are found in patients who have had invasion into the submucosa. Even so, the survival rate of this group averages about 93%. These figures should be considered in the light of the fact that, in Japan, about 30% of gastrectomies for cancer are carried out for early carcinoma. This means that the prognosis of gastric cancer can be very greatly improved if the disease is detected at an early stage of development. If this Japanese achievement is to be matched by European and North American workers then it is essential that we improve our methods of detection of early gastric cancer and make these facilities available to a much larger number of patients than hitherto.

CONCLUSION

All pathologists should become familiar with the Japanese classification of early gastric cancer. It is important in diagnosis and treatment as well as providing a firm basis for research into the histogenesis of carcinoma of the stomach.

Unless we adopt the meticulous techniques used by Japanese radiologists, endoscopists, and pathologists the yield of early gastric cancer in European and North American countries will remain low.

Carcinoma of the stomach is still a common form of malignant disease in North America and Europe and it has been shown that surgical treatment in the early stages gives excellent results in contrast to the very poor prognosis of advanced gastric cancer.

REFERENCES

1. Elster, K., Reiss, S. and Heinkel, K.: Histotopographische Unterschungen über die intestinale Metaplasie in Karzinom- und Ulkusmägen. *Z. Gesamte Inn. Med.* 15: 1053–1058, 1960.
2. Elster, K., Kolaczek, F., Shimamoto, K. and Freitag, H.: Early gastric cancer-experience in Germany. *Endoscopy* 7: 5–10, 1975.
3. Järvi, O., and Lauren, P.: On the role of heterotopias of the intestinal epithelium in the pathogenesis of gastric cancer. *Acta Pathol. Microbiol. Scand.* 29: 26–44, 1951.
4. Johansen, A. A.: Early gastric cancer. In *Monograph on Pathology of the Gastrointestinal Tract; Current Topics in Pathology,* edited by Morson, B. C., Berlin, Springer-Verlag. (To be published.)
5. Kidokoro, T.: Frequency of resection, metastasis and five-year survival rate of early gastric carcinoma in a surgical clinic. In *Gann Monograph on Cancer Research: Early Gastric Cancer,* edited by Murakami, T., Vol. 11, pp. 45–49. Baltimore, University Park Press, 1971.
6. Laurén, P.: The two histological main types of gastric carcinoma: diffuse and so-called

intestinal type carcinoma. An attempt at a histo-chemical classification. *Acta Pathol. Microbiol. Scand. 64:* 31–49, 1965.

7. Magnus, H. A.: Observations on the presence of intestinal epithelium in the gastric mucosa. *J. Pathol. Bacteriol. 44:* 389–398. 1937.

8. Morson, B. C.: Carcinoma arising from areas of intestinal metaplasia in the gastric mucosa. *Br. J. Cancer 9:* 377–385, 1955.

9. Morson B. C., Dawson, I. M. P.: *Gastrointestinal Pathology.* Oxford, Blackwell Scientific Publications, 1971.

10. Munoz, N., Correa, P., Cuello, C., and Duque, E.: Histologic type of gastric carcinoma in high and low risk areas. *Int. J. Cancer 3:* 809–818, 1968.

11. Murakami, T. (ed.): Early gastric cancer In *Gann Monograph on Cancer Research,* Vol. 11. Baltimore, University Park Press, 1971.

12. Muto, T., Bussey, H. J. R., and Morson, B. C.: The evolution of cancer of the colon and rectum. *Cancer 36:* 2251–2270, 1975.

13. Nagayo, T.: Mode of origin of gastric mucosal cancer with special reference to that of "superficial spreading type." In *Gann Monograph on Cancer Research: Epidemiological, Experimental and Clinical Studies on Gastric Cancer.* edited by Kinosita, R., Nagayo, T., Tanaka, T., pp 113–122. Tokyo, Maruzen Co., 1968.

14. Nakamura, K., Sugano, H., Maruyama, M., Sugiyama, N., and Takagi, K.: Histopathological study of primary locus of linitis plastica. *Stomach Intestine 10:* 79–86, 1975.

15. Nakamura, K., Sugano, H., and Takagi, K.: Carcinoma of the stomach in incipient phase, its histogenesis and histological appearances. *Gann 59.* 251–258, 1968.

16. Nakamura, K., Sugano, H., Takagi, K., and Fuchigami, A.: Histopathological study on early carcinoma of the stomach; some considerations on the ulcer-cancer by analysis of 144 foci of the superficial spreading carcinomas. *Gann 58:* 377–387, 1967.

17. Nakamura, K., Sugano, H., Takagi, K., and Kumakura, K.: Conception of histogenesis of gastric carcinoma. *Stomach Intestine 6:* 9–21, 1971.

18. Newcomb, W. D.: The relationship between peptic ulceration and gastric carcinoma. *Br. J. Surg. 20:* 279–308, 1932 and 1933.

19. Stout, A. P.: Superficial spreading type of carcinoma of the stomach. *Arch. Surg. 44:* 651–657, 1942.

Chapter 13

Lymphomas of the Gastrointestinal Tract

VINCENT J. MCGOVERN

Lymphomas frequently invade the alimentary tract or the mesentery from affected abdominal lymphnodes; less frequently they commence in the alimentary tract whence they invade adjacent organs or metastasize to other sites. This review is concerned with lymphomas commencing in the alimentary tract. Consequently it is necessary to restrict the material to those cases in which it is clear that there was no involvement beyond the alimentary tract and the associated lymphnodes of the affected portion. This eliminates advanced cases in which the alimentary tract is involved but in which it cannot be determined whether or not the lymphoma started in the alimentary tract.

Dawson, Cornes, and Morson[11] cited five criteria which they consider necessary to establish that a lymphoma in the intestinal tract is a primary growth. These same criteria are equally applicable to the stomach: (1.) There must be no palpable enlargement of superficial lymphnodes. (2.) Chest radiograms must show no mediastinal lymphnode enlargement. (3.) The white cell count, both total and differential, must be within normal limits. (4.) At laparotomy the alimentary lesion must predominate and any lymphnode involvement must be confined to those related to the involved area of gut. (5.) There must be no involvement of the liver or spleen.

Lymphomas of the alimentary tract are not common. Warren and Lulenski[55] found 28 (0.9%) among a total of 3132 gastrointestinal tumors.

Lymphomas of the alimentary tract occur mainly in persons in the 6th decade of life and older.[6, 19, 28, 31] Although they occur from time to time in young persons they are not common. However, lymphomas of the small intestine, though rare, are the commonest tumor of the gastrointestinal tract in childhood[17, 36] and they are often of well differentiated type. As Berg[6] pointed out, there is a bimodal distribution of intestinal lymphomas with one peak below the age of 10 years and the other averaging 53 years of age.

The stomach is usually more frequently affected by lymphomas than the remainder of the alimentary tract and in a composite series of 362 cases Berg[6] found that the stomach was involved in 51% of cases, the small intestine 33%, and the large intestine 16%. Naqvi, Burrows, and Kark[37] in their series of 162 cases also found that gastric lymphomas were more common than intestinal lymphomas and that lymphomas of the large intestine were distinctly rare.

TERMINOLOGY

At the present time the terminology of lymphomas, especially of the non-Hodgkin's lymphomas, has not been settled. Therefore, as a temporary measure, the following terminology is used for the non-Hodgkin's lymphomas: Follicular (nodular) or diffuse lymphoma (a.) well differentiated (lymphocytic, lymphosarcoma), (b.) moderate differentiation (lymphoblastic, mixed), (c.) poor differentiation (reticulum cell sarcoma) (Figs. 1–3).

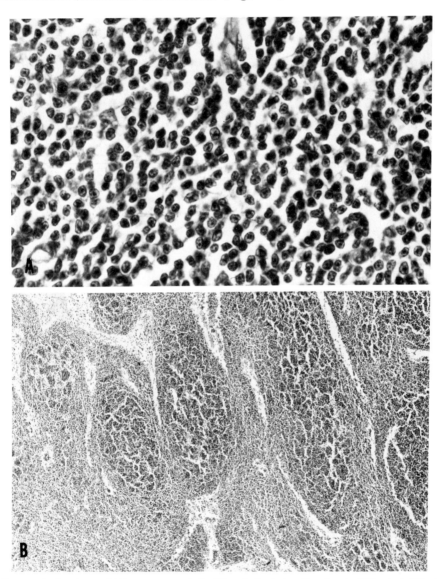

FIG. 1. *A*, female aged 77 years presented with pyloric obstruction due to diffusely infiltrating lymphoma. Histologically this was a fairly well differentiated tumor composed of small lymphocytic cells. Hematoxylin and eosin, × 300. *B*, the regional lymph nodes show follicular lymphoma. The follicles are poorly defined and have no germinal centers. Hematoxylin and eosin, × 48.

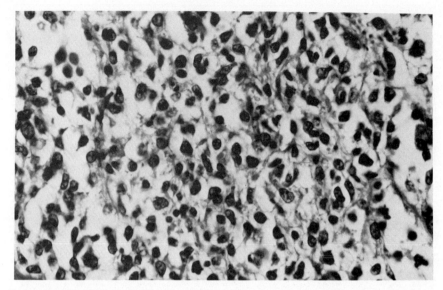

F<small>IG</small>. 2. Female aged 75 years presented with symptoms of peptic ulcer. She was found to have a prepyloric infiltrating lymphoma of intermediate differentiation. It is composed of cells of varying degrees of differentiation from lymphocytes to large poorly differentiated cells. Hematoxylin and eosin, × 300.

HISTOLOGIC DIAGNOSIS

The recognition of a lymphoma as opposed to a pseudolymphoma may be difficult.[11, 16, 26, 29,]   In differentiating tumor-like lymphoid hyperplasias from lymphomas one usually looks for follicles with germinal centers. Occasionally follicles are difficult to identify and an erroneous diagnosis of lymphoma may be made (Figs. 4, 5). In cases which seem to be lymphoma without lymphnode involvement one must always suspect the possibility of benign lymphoid hyperplasia. In the stomach these reactions usually accompany peptic ulceration, and consequently the finding of dense fibrosis with a breach in the muscularis propria should alert the pathologist to the possibility of benign lymphoid hyperplasia associated with chronic peptic ulceration.

Lymphomas of the gut are sometimes difficult to distinguish from carcinoma. When this happens, reticulin staining should prove helpful. Other helpful procedures are the demonstration of pyroninophilic granules in the cytoplasm of the neoplastic cells or in the case of carcinoma, the demonstration of mucin.

In the intestine small lymphoid polyps occur as a reactive phenomenon. In most cases the cause of these benign lymphoid polyps is unknown. They occur throughout the intestinal tract and in most cases present no diagnostic difficulty. Difficulty can arise however when there is follicular lymphoma which also may involve the entire alimentary tract. Here, the follicles have no germinal centers and in most cases the regional lymphnodes are also involved.

Most errors of diagnosis can be avoided by being aware that they occur.

LYMPHOMAS OF THE STOMACH

In the various published series of gastric neoplasms lymphomas comprise 1 to 5% of the total.[32, 9, 50] These are predominantly non-Hodgkin's lymphoma, the

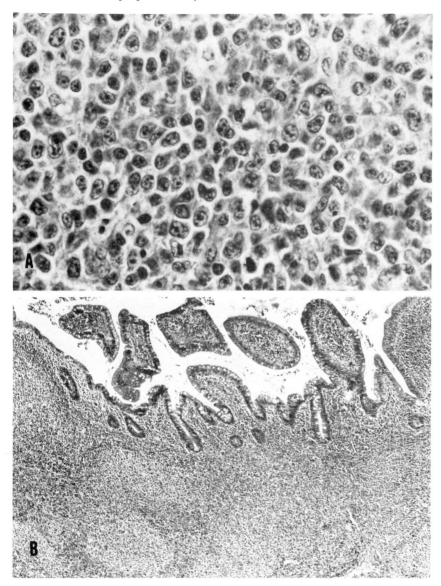

FIG. 3. *A*, female aged 37 years with obstruction of terminal ileum due to a sessile nodular tumor. The tumor is composed of large poorly differentiated cells. Hematoxylin and eosin, × 300. *B*, in some areas the follicular pattern of the lymphoma can still be discerned. Hematoxylin and eosin, × 48.

proportion of Hodgkin's disease varying up to 33%.[35] However, in most series Hodgkin's disease is much less common,[11, 2 , 31, 55] and in their review of 10 series of primary gastric lymphomas, Lee and Spratt[30] estimated that 3% of all malignant tumors of the stomach were lymphomas and that one-sixth (70 of 394) of these were Hodgkin's disease.

At Royal Prince Alfred Hospital (R. P. A. H.) 20 primary lymphomas of the stomach have been encountered among 965 malignant neoplasms seen in the 25

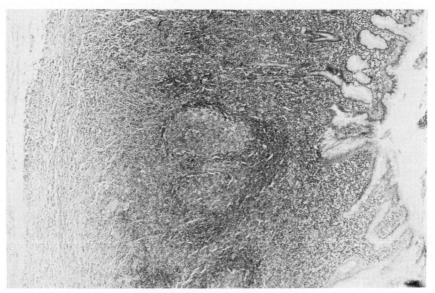

FIG. 4. Pseudo-lymphoma associated with a chronic peptic ulcer. Note the presence of lymphoid follicles with germinal centers. Hematoxylin and eosin, × 48.

years between 1951 and 1975, an incidence of little more than 2%. Of these, one was Hodgkin's disease.

AGE AND SEX

Most lymphomas of the stomach occur in persons of the 6th decade of life and older, and they are extremely rare in children.[17, 36] Males have a much higher incidence than females.

The patients seen at R. P. A. H. comprised 13 males and 7 females. The males ranged in age from 24 years to 73 years, 10 being more than 50 years of age and only 2 being under 40 years. Five of the 7 females ranged in age from 53 years to 77 years and the other two were 24 years and 46 years, respectively. The solitary patient with Hodgkin's disease of the stomach was a female aged 67 years.

PRESENTING SYMPTOMS[19, 28, 43]

Lymphomas of the stomach usually produce symptoms simulating peptic ulcer or carcinoma. Some are found to have a palpable mass. Hemorrhage, weight loss, and anorexia are less common symptoms. Among the R. P. A. H. patients 2 presented with dysphagia due to cardio-eosophageal obstruction, 2 with perforation, 2 with massive hematemesis, and 2 with pyloric obstruction. The remaining 12 presented because of ulcer-like pain.

DIAGNOSIS

In most cases of gastric lymphoma the diagnosis is made histologically from material obtained by laparotomy. Resection is a hazardous procedure and in view of the effectiveness of radiotherapy, only enough tissue for diagnosis alone may be all that is required.

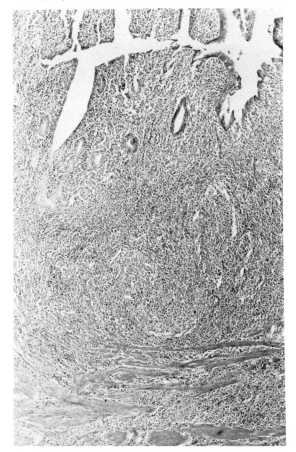

Fig. 5. Male 50 years of age with a large lymphoid mass around a chronic peptic ulcer. The lesion was biopsied and thought to be a lymphoma. He was treated with irradiation and at autopsy, 11 years later, there was no evidence of lymphoma. The lesion has been classified as a probable pseudo-lymphoma even though follicles are poorly developed. The only primitive cells are those in the ill-defined follicles. Elsewhere the cells are mature lymphocytes. The presence of a chronic peptic ulcer also raises doubts as to whether this was a true lymphoma. Hematoxylin and eosin, × 48.

Gastric biopsy with modern gastroscopes is a very useful way of diagnosing gastric cancer including lymphoma. In doubtful cases mucus stains help to identify carcinoma cells and methyl green pyronin stains will often demonstrate pyroninophilia in lymphoma cells. In the case of well differentiated lymphomas it may not be possible in very small biopsies to determine whether or not lymphoma is present.

Cytologic examination of gastric washings is a very accurate method of diagnosis.[43] The doubtful case is treated in the same way as doubtful biopsies.

RADIOLOGIC APPEARANCE[27, 47, 49, 51, 52]

The distinction between lymphoma of the stomach and carcinoma cannot be made with certainty, nor on occasions can it be distinguished from benign ulcer.

A large ulcerated mass which does not reduce the volume of the stomach, large rugae leading to an ulcer, or a mass with several craters are all features which are very suggestive, though not absolutely diagnostic, of lymphoma.

GROSS APPEARANCE

The usual surgical diagnosis that accompanies the resected specimen to the laboratory is carcinoma and it comes as something of a surprise to the surgeon to find that the tumor was a lymphoma.

Lymphomas of the stomach may be diffusely infiltrative or raised and plaque-like with ulceration of the surface (Figs. 6, 7). They occur most frequently in the prepyloric region. Polypoid lesions occur but are uncommon and giant rugosities are distinctly rare.[14] One of the R. P. A. H. tumors projected into the gastric

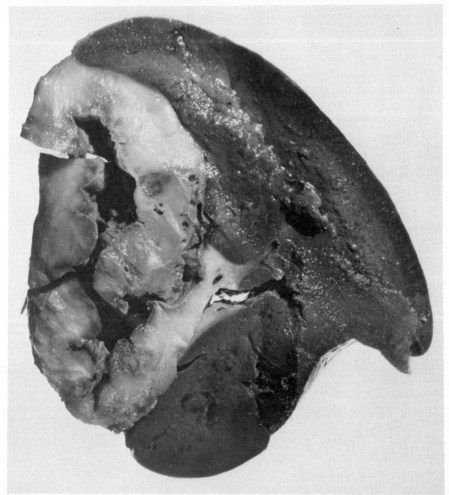

FIG. 6. Female aged 23 years, 24 weeks pregnant, was admitted to hospital with massive hematemesis. She died postoperatively. An infiltrating tumor involving most of the stomach was found. It was adherent to the spleen but not infiltrating it. The tumor was a lymphoma of mixed cells, *i.e.*, intermediate differentiation.

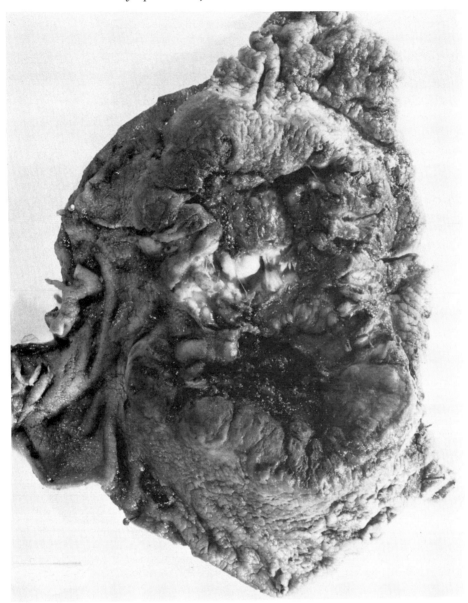

FIG. 7. Male of 56 years with peptic ulcer symptoms. A portion of stomach with a large ulcerating raised neoplastic plaque was resected. It was composed of large poorly differentiated cells and lymphnodes were involved. The patient died from operative complications a month later.

cavity like a cauliflower while another had multiple nodules in the stomach wall; the remainder were infiltrative and ulcerated. Lymphoma of the stomach tends to penetrate the stomach wall and to perforate,[39] or occasionally, as observed in two R. P. A. H. patients, to infiltrate adjacent structures such as the anterior abdominal wall or the transverse colon.

MICROSCOPIC APPEARANCE

Any of the varieties of lymphoma may be found in the stomach, the majority presenting no great difficulty in diagnosis (Table 1). There are occasions, however, when the distinction between lymphoma and pseudo-lymphoma and between lymphoma and carcinoma is difficult. This problem has been discussed above.

Apart from the main mass of tumor, multicentric foci occur in the lamina propria of the mucosa with or without submucosal involvement in more than half of the cases.[6]

In the large series of Loehr et al.[31] and also in that of Naqvi, Burrows, and Kark[37] well differentiated lymphoma (small cell lymphosarcoma) was the commonest while Hodgkin's disease was the least common, occurring in 6 of 63 cases and 2 of 116 cases, respectively.

Among the R. P. A. H. cases (Table 1) there were three for which histologic material was no longer available. They had been diagnosed as "reticulum cell sarcoma".

TABLE 1. LYMPHOMAS OF STOMACH

Histologic type	No. cases
Follicular, well differentiated	1
Diffuse, well differentiated	2
Diffuse, moderately differentiated	6
Diffuse, poorly differentiated	7
Hodgkin's disease, mixed cellularity	1
Reticulum cell sarcoma[a]	3
Total	20

[a] Histologic material not available for review.

Lymphnode involvement is usually found in lymphoma of the stomach and was demonstrated in the case of Hodgkin's disease and in 15 of the 19 non-Hodgkin's lymphomas.

TREATMENT

Wolferth et al.[5] found that when curative surgery for lymphoma of the stomach was able to be carried out, i.e., no lymphnode involvement, postoperative irradiation was unnecessary. If lymphnodes were found to be involved or if the gastric lesion was inoperable they recommended irradiation and 2 of their patients with inoperable tumors survived more than 7 years. Seven of 15 eligible patients survived more than 5 years.

The first published series of patients with gastric lymphoma submitted to surgery and then radiotherapy was that of Crile, Hazard, and Allen,[10] who had 68% with an average period of survival of 5 years. Since then the general consensus of opinion has been that surgery and postoperative radiotherapy should lead to 5-year survivals of 40% or more.[3, 1, 5] The postoperative death rate, however, is high.

Radiotherapeutic techniques have improved greatly in the last few years and as in our own experience simple palliative or diagnostic surgery followed by radiotherapy may result in long-term survival.

PROGNOSIS

The prognosis of gastric lymphomas depends upon the type of lymphoma. Hodgkin's disease has a lower 5-year survival rate than the other lymphomas. Marshall and Adamson[34] found that 27% of patient with Hodgkin's disease of the stomach survived 5 years against 39% for the other lymphomas. Dawson, Cornes, and Morson[11] in their review of 117 cases of gastric lymphoma found 22 examples of Hodgkin's disease, of which 7 survived more than 5 years. Most reports of gastric lymphomas contain few cases of Hodgkin's disease and consequently their statistics are not significant. It is clear, however, that Hodgkin's disease of the stomach is potentially curable though the survival figures are not as good as for other forms of lymphoma.

In non-Hodgkin's lymphoma survival rates depend upon the type of lymphoma. Follicular lymphomas have much better survival rates than diffuse lymphomas. Apart from this, well differentiated lymphocytic lymphomas have 5-year survival rates in the various published series that vary between 83% and 100%, and what used to be called reticulum cell sarcoma has between 36% and 50% 5-year survival.[6, 19, 31, 37, , 51]

Lymphnode involvement does not seem to alter the prognosis to any significant degree.[11]

Among the R. P. A. H. cases there were 7 postoperative deaths. In each case there had been resection of the affected portion of stomach. Those who survived operation had a relatively good prognosis even when the neoplasm had not been entirely removed.

TABLE 2. LYMPHOMAS OF THE STOMACH

Type	No. Cases
Total no. patients	20
Died postoperatively	5
Eligible for 5-year survival	6
5-Year survivals	4
Total lymphoma deaths (including postoperative deaths)	9
Died from other causes	2
Number now alive	7
Lost to follow-up 2 and 4 years after diagnosis	2

From Table 2 it can be seen that 4 of the 6 eligible patients have survived 5 years or longer, and that the greatest hazard was the surgical operation.

TABLE 3. LYMPHOMAS OF THE STOMACH: FIVE-YEAR SURVIVORS

Case	Sex	Age	Type	Lymph Node Involvement	Survival	Treatment
1	M	?	Mod. diff.	+	11 yrs.	Incomplete resection + irradiation
2	M	59	Poor. diff.	−	9 yrs.	Resection + irradiation
3	M	58	Poor. diff.	+	8 yrs.	Resection + irradiation (transverse colon involved)
4	F	46	Mod. diff.	?	6 yrs.	Resection + irradiation

As noted by Berg,[6] perforation of the stomach is likely to be followed by death of the patient. Apart from surgical considerations, the single most important pathologic feature in assessing prognosis is the type of tumor, but in the individual case other factors come into play. As can be seen in Table 3, a patient with involvement of the transverse colon by a tumor of poor differentiation with lymphnode involvement is still alive and well 8 years after resection and postoperative irradiation.

Five R. P. A. H. patients who survived the postoperative period died within 5 years. One of these who was treated by irradiation after laparotomy and biopsy without resection had no demonstrable tumor at postmortem examination 1 year later, even though the tumor had involved the anterior abdominal wall. One had progressive disease and died from cerebral involvement 3 years after diagnosis. The remaining 3 patients died from progressive disease in shorter periods despite irradiation.

LYMPHOMAS OF THE SMALL INTESTINE

Lymphomas form up to one-half of primary malignant tumors of the small intestine.[39, 5, 56] However there are interesting geographic differences in incidence. In the Middle East, malignant lymphomas of the small intestine are relatively common. Al-Khateeb[2] of Iraq found that 8.7% of all gastrointestinal tumors were primary lymphomas of the small intestine compared with the 0.9% of 3132 gastrointestinal tumors found by Warren and Lulenski[55] in the United States.

Tumors of the duodenum are less common than tumors of the jejunum and ileum and those of the ileum are mainly in the terminal portion. Berg[6] in a composite series of 362 gastrointestinal lymphomas found that 33% occurred in the small intestine. The majority of these involved the ileum and the least common site was the duodenum. Loehr *et al.*[31] reported 25 small intestine cases, of which 4 were in the duodenum, 12 in the jejunum, and 9 in the ileum.

There were 16 primary lymphomas of the small intestine among 50 malignant neoplasms at R. P. A. H., an incidence of 32%. Of these 6 were primary lymphomas of the jejunum and 10 were in the ileum. In the same period there were 6 primary malignant tumors of other types in the jejunum and 7 in the ileum.

Among the R. P. A. H. cases there was none with a lymphoma confined to the duodenum diagnosed during life. There had been 1 case in which follicular lymphoma, affecting the entire intestinal tract from duodenum to rectum, was an incidental finding at postmortem examination but this case is not included in the series. Furthermore, 2 cases in which the tumors were situated in the duodenojejunal region were classified as jejunal because they were predominantly in that portion of the small intestine.

AGE AND SEX

Lymphomas of the small intestine occur in the same age group as do lymphomas of the stomach except that there is also a peak in the incidence in children.[36] Kahn,[28] however, found that his 24 adult cases were between 20 and 52 years of age, with a mean age of 36 years. There were 14 males and 10 females. In the Middle East lymphomas occur at an earlier age among Arabs, Israelis, and non-European Jews. Eidelman, Parkins, and Rubin[13] reported 9 cases in which there was lymphoma of the small intestine associated with steatorrhea. Their average age was 21 years.

Six of the R. P. A. H. series of 16 primary lymphomas of the small intestine occurred in males and 10 in females. The age incidence ranged from 28 to 70 years for males and 23 to 77 years for females. As with lymphomas of the stomach, they occurred predominantly in the older age groups, 5 of the males and 7 of the 10 females being more than 50 years of age.

PRESENTING SYMPTOMS

The commonest manifestation of lymphoma of the small intestine is pain of obstructive type with or without the other manifestations of obstruction, consisting of nausea, vomiting, anorexia, and change in bowel habits.[3, 11, 33] In about one-third of cases a mass can be felt in the abdomen.[28] Irvine and Johnstone[25] reported 17 cases of non-Hodgkin's primary lymphoma of the bowel in which perforation was the first evidence of disease in 8 cases. Perforation occurred more commonly in the less well differentiated tumors.

Intussusception tends to occur when the tumors form a nodule protruding into the intestinal lumen.[7, 17]

Lymphoma of the duodenum may involve the ampulla of Vater and cause obstructive jaundice as it did in 3 of Warren's 4 cases.[53]

MALABSORPTION SYNDROME

Among cases reported by Kahn, Selzer, and Kaschula[28] there were 8 in which the presenting symptoms were those of malabsorption. The average duration of the symptoms of malabsorption prior to the diagnosis of lymphoma was 3 years. A sprue-like syndrome may complicate lymphoma of the gut or lymphoma, either Hodgkin's, or non-Hodgkin's lymphoma, may commence in the intestine of a patient with gluten enteropathy.[8, 17, 24] When Fairlie and Mackie[15] first described steatorrhea in association with abdominal lymphomas they ascribed the condition to obstruction of mesenteric lymphatics.[12] However, patients with lymphoma of the small intestine may have villous atrophy in areas unaffected by the lymphoma even in the absence of malabsorption. Dutz *et al*[12] found areas of flat mucosa in 15% of small intestines at autopsy in nonlymphomatous cases, and in 90% of patients with intestinal lymphoma. They concluded that sprue-like villous atrophy was a trigger-like factor in its development.

Malabsorption is very common among patients with intestinal lymphoma in the Middle East. Eidelman, Parkins, and Rubin[13] were the first to describe this entity of which the salient features are young males with malabsorption, abdominal pain, and clubbing of the fingers.[1, 4, 13] Ramot[42] emphasizes that intestinal lymphoma is common among non-European (Sephardic) Jews but among European (Askenazic) Jews the incidence is similar to that in non-Jews elsewhere. Most of the cases have been non-Hodgkin's lymphoma but malabsorption has been recorded in Hodgkin's disease also.[8, 24]

There are other ethnic groups in which the combination of lymphoma and steatorrhea exist, and Novis *et al.*[38] recorded 22 cases of lymphoma presenting with steatorrhea. Their ages ranged from 19 to 57 years, the majority being under 30 years. The disorder they describe is very similar to the Mediterranean type of lymphoma and since it occurs most frequently in the Cape Blacks of South Africa they regard this term as a misnomer.

Paraproteinemia

In addition to malabsorption, patients with primary lymphoma in the Middle East sometimes exhibit paraproteinemia. Rambaud *et al.*[41] in 1968 described α-heavy chain disease occurring in a patient with mediterranean type of abdominal lymphoma. Since then there have been other reports of this combination. Shahid *et al.*[46] have described 5 cases in which there was abdominal pain, diarrhea, weight loss, and malabsorption. The subject of malabsorption in association with intestinal lymphomas is reviewed by Lee and Spratt.[30]

Thirteen of the 16 R. P. A. H. cases presented because of abdominal pain. Two of the other three presented with perforation and one with volvulus of the affected loop of the ileum.

Lymphomas associated with steatorrhea occurred in two patients, a male aged 35 years and a female of 33 years. The female patient had been known to have gluten enteropathy before the onset of the lymphoma, but in the other patient steatorrhea had not been documented prior to the onset of obstructive symptoms.

Diagnosis

The diagnosis of small bowel lymphoma is usually made on histologic examination of the resected specimen. However, it should be possible in some cases to make a positive diagnosis by mucosal biopsies of the duodenum and jejunum. Five of the cases of Novis *et al.*[38] were diagnosed by this procedure. Lesions of the cecal region and the terminal ileum should be accessible to the colonoscope.

Radiologic Appearance

There are no specific radiologic findings, except that when the pattern in barium studies of patients with celiac disease is combined with obstruction, lymphoma may be suspected. Apart from this, radiologic studies will merely reflect the gross morphology of the lesion. When there is an infiltrating tumor of the terminal ileum the appearances may suggest Crohn's disease.

Gross Appearance

Faulkner and Dockerty[17] described the lesions of intestinal lymphoma as ulcerative, aneurysmal, and polypoid. Dawson, Cornes, and Morson[11] have 4 categories: bulky protuberant, annular, aneurysmal, and polypoid. Our experience is more in keeping with the latter. Bulky protuberant tumors are tumors which are likely to cause intussusception. Annular lesions at first glance are sometimes difficult to recognize as neoplastic. They are ulcerated, frequently multiple, and cause narrowing of the lumen of the gut. In aneurysmal lesions the lymphoma infiltrates the wall of the gut causing it to be thickened and rather firm. Nevertheless the diameter of the lumen both proximally and distally is rather less than that of the aneurysmal part.

Among the R. P. A. H. cases there were 6 with lymphomas of the small intestine appearing as solitary nodules which caused obstructive symptoms

(Fig. 8). In 4 there were multiple constricting annular tumors, which were recurrent over a period of 6 years in the one male with steatorrhea, until his death (Figs. 9, 10). There were 3 patients with segments of bowel infiltrated by lymphoma, *i.e.,* aneurysmal lesions, two of whom presented with perforation and one with volvulus. In a postmortem case follicular lymphoma extending from the duodenum to rectum was an incidental finding. This case is not included here.

MICROSCOPIC APPEARANCE

The histologic types of lymphoma are summarized in Table 4. There were no examples of Hodgkin's disease.

The histologic types do not show the preponderance of well differentiated tumors seen in other published series, but this may be due to the series being too

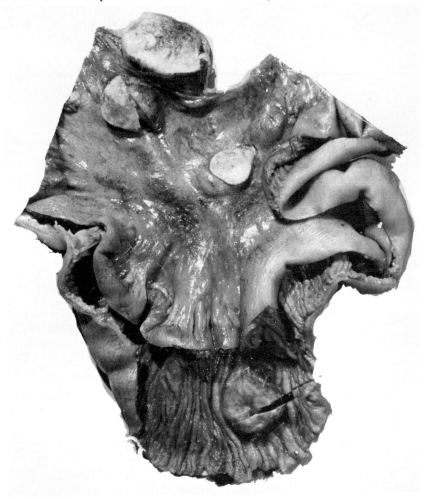

FIG. 8. Female aged 37 years with symptoms of obstruction of the terminal ileum. There is a raised nodular tumor in the intestine and large regional lymph nodes. The microscopic appearances are illustrated in Figure 3. The patient is still alive and well 8 months postoperatively.

TABLE 4. LYMPHOMAS OF SMALL INTESTINE

Histological type		Lymph node involvement	
		(+)	(−)
Follicular			
Moderately differentiated	1	1	
Poorly differentiated	1	1	
Diffuse			
Well differentiated	2		
Moderately differentiated	6	3	2
Poorly differentiated	6	3	1

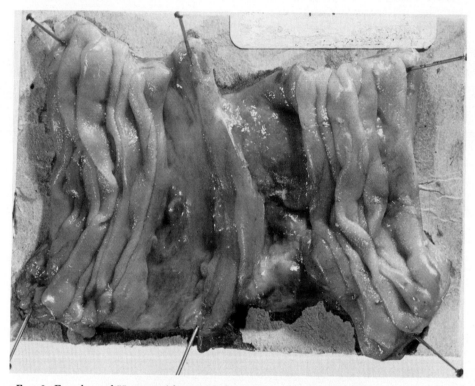

FIG. 9. Female aged 55 years with an encircling ulcerated tumor of terminal ileum composed of cells of intermediate differentiation. Lymph nodes were not involved. The patient was lost to follow-up, having in the meantime developed a carcinoma of the breast.

small to be representative. Lymphnodes were available for examination in 11 cases, of which 8 contained tumor.

Microscopically lymphomas of the small intestine differ from those of the stomach in that they commence in the submucosa and the overlying mucosa eventually ulcerates, whereas gastric lymphomas seem to start in the lamina propria of the mucosa itself.

TREATMENT

The usual treatment is resection, including the relevant lymphnodes. Fu and Perzin[20] reported 26 examples of primary intestinal lymphoma and they recom-

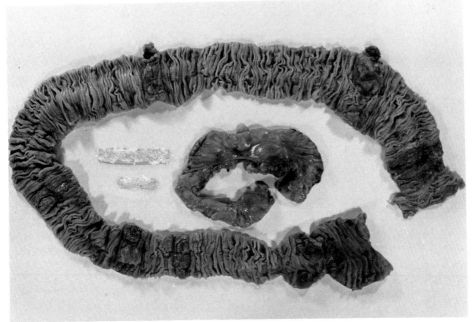

F<small>IG</small>. 10. Male aged 35 years with multiple lesions of jejunum. There were subsequent recurrences after 3 years and the patient died 6 years after the initial resection. He developed the malabsorption syndrome and was found to have flattened intestinal mucosa.

mend that there be wide segmental resection including the contiguous lymphnodes. They recommend radiotherapy if the following unfavorable signs are present: lymphnode involvement, incomplete resection, perforation, fistula, and multicentric tumors. Cures by radiotherapy alone have been reported.[no yk]

All of the cases at R. P. A. H. were treated by resection and radiotherapy was given to 4.

P<small>ROGNOSIS</small>

The 5-year-survival figure of Loehr *et al.*[31] for lymphoma of the small intestine was 40% compared with 53% for gastric lymphomas. Faulkner and Dockerty[17] however, had only 3 (21%) 5-year survivals among 14 eligible patients.

The survival rate in large series can be correlated with cell type. Dawson, Cornes, and Morson,[11] in a review of 176 cases of primary lymphoma of the gut, found that 50% of patients with follicular lymphoma, 25% with lymphosarcoma, and 10% with reticulum cell sarcoma survived 5 years. Only one-half of these 5-year survivors, however, lived 10 years or more after treatment.

Among the R. P. A. H. patients (Table 5) there were 12 eligible for 5-year survivorship, of whom only 1 survived free of disease, a female of 23 years who had a volvulus involving a loop of ileum in which there was a diffuse infiltrating poorly differentiated lymphoma. This patient is alive and well more than 25 years since resection of the tumor. Another patient, a male aged 35 years, survived 6 years with recurrent tumors of the jejunum. His tumor was of moderate differentiation. Two of the patients with progressive disease had well differentiated tumors and 3 had tumors of moderate differentiation.

TABLE 5. SURVIVAL RATES FOR LYMPHOMAS OF SMALL INTESTINE

Total no. patients	16
Died postoperatively	5
Eligible for 5-year survival	7
Survived 5 years free of disease	1
Survived 5 years with recurrent disease	1
Total deaths	11
Number now alive	3
Lost to follow-up	2

As with lymphoma of the stomach, there are no features upon which one can give a confident prognosis in the individual case. All deaths that were not postoperative were, in the R. P. A. H. series, due to progressive disease. However, it has been stated that the prognosis is worse in patients with malabsorption. Cornes, Wallace, and Morson[9] stated that lymphomas associated with steatorrhea had a higher proportion of Hodgkin's disease, that the tumors tended to be multiple often in the jejunum and proximal ileum, and that despite surgical removal, fresh lesions developed, with an eventual fatal outcome. This was in accordance with our experience.

LYMPHOMAS OF THE LARGE INTESTINE

Primary appendiceal or colonic lymphomas are rare. Warren and Lulenski[55] found that only 0.3% of 2510 colonic and rectal cancers were lymphomatous. Pseudo-lymphomas, however, especially in the rectum, are very much more common.[9, 37]

The commonest site for lymphoma is the cecal region and less frequently the rectosigmoid area. They can occur in any part of the large intestine including the appendix and are commonly multiple.[3, 5, 7, 22, 31, 54, 57, 59]

AGE AND SEX

The number of cases reported is so small that all one can say is that there is perhaps a greater incidence in males and that although lymphomas of the large intestine occur at any age, the majority of patients are over the age of 50 years, though Lee and Spratt[30] had one patient aged 4 years.

PRESENTING SYMPTOMS

The symptoms of lymphoma of the large intestine are much the same as for carcinoma, consisting of abdominal pain, weight loss, rectal bleeding, and change in bowel habits.[22, 57, 59] There is an association with chronic ulcerative colitis. Two of Warren's[53] 8 patients with malignant lymphoma of the rectum also had long-standing ulcerative colitis and Dawson, Cornes, and Morson[11] encountered 7 patients with lymphoma complicating chronic ulcerative colitis.

DIAGNOSIS

The diagnosis of lymphomas of the large intestine can only be made histologically. Now that the colonoscope is available biopsy specimens can be obtained from the more remote parts of the colon which were not accessible to the sigmoidoscope and lesions that were once occult can now be revealed.

RADIOLOGIC APPEARANCE

As with lymphomas in other parts of the alimentary tract there are no specific appearances. Features favoring malignant lymphoma are longer segmental involvement, dilatation of the gut, and flattening of the mucosal surface.[57] While the x-rays may be abnormal, the diagnosis of lymphoma is unlikely to be the first choice in the differential diagnosis.

GROSS APPEARANCE

Lymphomas of the large intestine are similar to those of the small intestine but circumscribed tumors projecting into the lumen are most commonly found (Fig. 11) and annular lesions are uncommon. Infiltrating tumors may penetrate pericolic tissues. As in the small intestine the tumors may be multiple.

In cases of follicular lymphoma there may be a diffuse polyposis. These polyps differ from adenoma in having a smooth mucosa-covered surface instead of the lobulated pattern that characterizes adenoma. Lymphomas of the rectosigmoid region are rare and have to be distinguished from benign lymphoid polyps which are much more common.[23] The distinction should not be very difficult although there is always the possibility that a lymphoma with a follicular pattern can be mistaken for a benign lesion. The histologic features of benign lymphoid polyps of the rectum and their distinction from lymphomas are well described by Helwig and Hansen.[23]

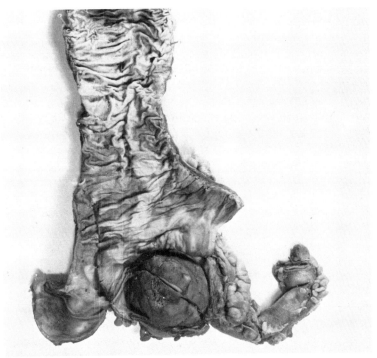

FIG. 11. Male aged 62 years with a polypoid lymphoma of the cecum, composed of cells of intermediate differentiation. Lymphnodes were not involved. After 9 years of freedom from disease the patient developed a carcinoma of the stomach which could not be resected.

Three lymphomas of the large intestine have been seen at R. P. A. H. Two were polypoid lesions in the cecum and one was an infiltrating tumor of the ascending colon which penetrated into the pericolic tissues.

MICROSCOPIC APPEARANCE

Lymphomas of the large intestine are similar to those elsewhere in the alimentary tract. Both Hodgkin's disease and non-Hodgkin's lymphomas occur.

TREATMENT

The ideal treatment is surgical resection and if there is doubt about completeness of the excision or if lymphnodes are involved, it is usual to give postoperative irradiation. [0, 59]

PROGNOSIS

The prognosis is relatively good in that a 5-year survival of 55% or better and a 10-year figure of 50% can be expected.[22, 59] Perry, Cross, and Morson, [0] reporting from St. Mark's Hospital (London), found that of their 22 patients with rectal lymphomas, 3 were Hodgkin's disease, 4 were reticulum cell sarcomas, and 15 were lymphosarcomas. Eight of the 10 patients treated by chemotherapy or radiotherapy alone died shortly afterwards. Of those who had radiotherapy after sigmoid colostomy 2 were alive and well. Nine had surgical procedures, 8 by abdominoperineal resection and 1 by intrapelvic exenteration. Five of these survived.

Our own experience is very small, consisting as it does of 3 patients. One, a female of 69 years, presented with pain and a palpable mass in the right iliac fossa. She was found to have a polypoid tumor in the cecum which was resected. The lesion was a non-Hodgkin's lymphoma of intermediate malignancy with lymphnode involvement. She died after 3 years from progressive disease despite radiotherapy. The second patient was a male aged 62 years who had a polypoid lymphoma of intermediate differentiation in his cecum. This was resected. Lymphnodes were not involved and the patient lived 9 years free of symptoms until he developed a carcinoma of the stomach which proved inoperable. The third patient, a recent admission to the hospital, was a male aged 54 years with an infiltrating lymphoma of the ascending colon which had penetrated into the pericolic tissues. It was a fairly well differentiated tumor with a follicular pattern. The tumor was inoperable and is to be treated by radiotherapy.

SUMMARY

Lymphomas occurring primarily in the alimentary tract present in the same way as carcinomas. Because they have a much better prognosis than carcinoma, especially in the case of gastric lymphomas, it is important that they be diagnosed. For this reason, laparotomy if necessary should be undertaken in order to establish a histologic diagnosis of all alimentary neoplasms. With modern equipment, however, it is often possible to obtain enough tissue for diagnosis by endoscopic means. The ideal treatment is surgery, but if there is doubt about the completeness of excision or if there are involved lymphnodes, postoperative radiotherapy is desirable.

The types of primary alimentary lymphoma are similar to those occurring in lymphnodes, and they may be follicular (nodular) or diffuse. Hodgkin's disease is less common than the other lymphomas and has a somewhat worse prognosis. The main prognostic features of alimentary lymphomas are type of lymphoma and degree of differentiation. Follicular lymphomas have a better prognosis than diffuse lymphomas and well differentiated lymphocytic lesions have a better prognosis than large cell poorly differentiated tumors. Lymphnode involvement has no significance in the overall survival rates.

REFERENCES

1. al-Bahrani, Z. R., and Bakir, F.: Primary intestinal lymphoma. A challenging problem in abdominal pain. *Ann. R. Coll. Surg. Engl. 49:* 103–113, 1971.
2. Al-Khateeb, A. K.: Primary malignant lymphoma of the small intestine. *Int. Surg. 54:* 295–300, 1970.
3. Allen, A. W., Donaldson, G., Sniffen, R. C., and Goodale, F.: Primary malignant lymphoma of the gastro-intestinal tract. *Ann. Surg. 140:* 428–438, 1954.
4. al-Saleem, T., and al-Bahrani, Z.: Malignant lymphoma of the small intestine in Iraq (Middle East lymphoma). *Cancer 31:* 291–294, 1973.
5. Azzopardi, J. G., and Menzies, T.: Primary malignant lymphoma of the alimentary tract. *Br. J. Surg. 47:* 358–366, 1960.
6. Berg, J. W.: Primary lymphomas of the human gastrointestinal tract. *Natl. Cancer Inst. Monogr. 32:* 211–220, 1969.
7. Burman, S. O., and van Wyk, F. A. K.: Lymphomas of the small intestine and cecum. *Ann. Surg. 143:* 349–359, 1956.
8. Cornes, J. S.: Hodgkin's disease of the gastrointestinal tract. *Proc. R. Soc. Med. 60:* 732–733, 1967.
9. Cornes, J. S., Wallace, M. H., and Morson, B. C.: Benign lymphomas of the rectum and anal canal; a study of 100 cases. *J. Pathol. Bacteriol. 82:* 371–382, 1961.
10. Crile, G., Hazard, J. B., Allen, K. L.: Primary lymphosarcoma of the stomach. *Ann. Surg. 135:* 39–43, 1952.
11. Dawson, I. M. P., Cornes, J. S., and Morson, B. C.: Primary malignant lymphoid tumours of the intestinal tract; report of 37 cases with a study of factors influencing prognosis. *Br. J. Surg. 49:* 80–89, 1961.
12. Dutz, W., Asvadi, S., Sadri, S., and Kohout, E.: Intestinal lymphoma and sprue; a systematic approach. *Gut 12:* 804–810, 1971.
13. Eidelman, S., Parkins, R. A., and Rubin, C. E.: Abdominal lymphoma presenting as malabsorption; a clinico-pathologic study of nine cases in Israel and a review of the literature. *Medicine 45:* 111–137, 1966.
14. Ellis, H. A., and Lannigan, R.: Primary lymphoid neoplasms of the stomach. *Gut 4:* 145–152, 1963.
15. Fairlie, N. H., and Mackie, F. P.: The clinical and biochemical syndrome in lymphadenoma and allied diseases involving the mesenteric lymph glands. *Br. Med. J. 1:* 375–380, 1937.
16. Faris, T. D., and Saltzstein, S. L.: Gastric lymphoid hyperplasia; a lesion confused with lymphosarcoma. *Cancer 17:* 207–212, 1964.
17. Faulkner, J. W., and Dockerty, M. B.: Lymphosarcoma of the small intestine. *Surg. Gynecol. Obstet. 95:* 76–84, 1952.
18. Frazer, J. W.: Malignant lymphomas of the gastrointestinal tract. *Surg. Gynecol. Obstet. 108:* 182–190, 1959.
19. Friedman, A. I.: Primary lymphosarcoma of the stomach; a clinical study of seventy-five cases. *Am. J. Med. 26:* 783–796, 1959.
20. Fu, Y.-S., and Perzin, K. H.: Lymphosarcoma of the small intestine; a clinicopathologic study. *Cancer 29:* 645–659, 1972.
21. Fu, K., and Stewart, J. R.: Radiotherapeutic management of small intestinal lymphoma with malabsorption. *Cancer 31:* 286–290, 1973.

22. Glick, D. D., and Soule, E. H.: Primary malignant lymphoma of colon or appendix; report of 27 cases. *Arch. Surg. 92:* 144–151, 1966.

23. Helwig, E. B., and Hansen, J.: Lymphoid polyps (benign lymphoma) and malignant lymphoma of the rectum and anus. *Surg. Gynecol. Obstet. 92:* 233–243, 1951.

24. Hoskins, E. O. L.: Unusual radiological manifestations of Hodgkin's disease. *Proc. R. Soc. Med. 60:* 729–732, 1967.

25. Irvine, W. T., and Johnstone, J. M.: Lymphosarcoma of the small intestine; with special reference to perforating tumours. *Br. J. Surg. 42:* 611–618, 1955.

26. Jacobs, D. S.: Primary gastric malignant lymphoma and pseudolymphoma. *Am. J. Clin. Pathol. 40:* 379–394, 1963.

27. Joseph, J. I., and Lattes, R.: Gastric lymphosarcoma; clinico-pathologic analysis of 71 cases and its relation to disseminated lymphosarcoma. *Am. J. Clin. Pathol. 45:* 653–669, 1966.

28. Kahn, L. B., Selzer, G., Kaschula, R. O. C.: Primary gastrointestinal lymphoma; a clinicopathologic study of fifty-seven cases. *Am. J. Dig. Dis. 17:* 219–232, 1972.

29. Kay, S.: Lymphoid tumors of the stomach. *Surg. Gynecol. Obstet. 118:* 1059–1066, 1964.

30. Lee, Yeu-Tsu N., and Spratt, J. S.: Malignant lymphoma; Nodal and Extranodal Diseases. New York, Grune & Stratton, 1974.

31. Loehr, W. J., Mujahed, Z., Zahn, F. D., Gray, G. F., and Thorbjarnarson, B.: Primary lymphoma of the gastrointestinal tract; a review of 100 cases. *Ann. Surg. 170:* 232–238, 1969.

32. McNeer, G., and Berg, J. W.: The clinical behavior and management of primary malignant lymphoma of the stomach. *Surgery 46:* 829–840, 1959.

33. Marcuse, P. M., Stout, A. P.: Primary lymphosarcoma of the small intestine; analysis of thirteen cases and review of the literature. *Cancer 3:* 459–474, 1950.

34. Marshall, S. F., and Adamson, N. E.: Sarcoma of the stomach; tumors of lymphatic and reticuloendothelial origin (62 cases). *Surg. Clin. North. Am. 39:* 711–718, 1959.

35. Marshall, S. F., and Brown, L.: Primary malignant lymphoid tumors of the stomach. *Surg. Clin. North Am. 30:* 885–892, 1950.

36. Mestel, A. L.: Lymphosarcoma of the small intestine in infancy and childhood. *Ann. Surg. 149:* 87–94, 1959.

37. Naqvi, M. S., Burrows, L., and Kark, A. E.: Lymphoma of the gastrointestinal tract; prognostic guides based on 162 cases. *Ann. Surg. 170:* 221–231, 1969.

38. Novis, B. H., Banks, S., Marks, I. N., Selzer, G., Kahn, L., and Sealy, R.: Abdominal lymphoma presenting with malabsorption. *Q. J. Med. 40:* 521–540, 1971.

39. Pagtalunan, R. J. G., Mayo, C. W., and Dockerty, M. B.: Primary malignant tumors of the small intestine. *Am. J. Surg. 108:* 13–18, 1964.

40. Perry, P. M., Cross, R. M., Morson, B. C.: Primary malignant lymphoma of the rectum (22 cases). *Proc. R. Soc. Med. 65:* 72, 1972.

41. Rambaud, J. C., Bognel, C., Prost, A., Bernier, J. L., Le Quintrec, Y., Lambling, A., Dannon, F., Hurez, D., and Seligmann, M.: Clinico-pathological study of a patient with "Mediterranean" type of abdominal lymphoma and a new type of IgA abnormality ("alpha chain disease"). *Digestion 1:* 321–336, 1968.

42. Ramot, B.: Intestinal lymphoma with malabsorption in Mediterranean populations. *Isr. J. Med. Sci. 7:* 1488–1490, 1971.

43. Rubin, C. E. and Massey, B. W.: The preoperative diagnosis of gastric and duodenal malignant lymphoma by exfoliative cytology. *Cancer 7:* 271–288, 1954.

44. Saltzstein, S. L.: Extranodal malignant lymphomas and pseudolymphomas. In *Pathology Annual 1969,* edited by Sommers, S. C., pp. 159–184. New York, Appleton-Century-Crofts, 1969.

45. Schmutzer, K. J., Holleran, W. M., and Regan, J. F.: Tumors of the small bowel. *Am. J. Surg. 108:* 270–276, 1964.

46. Shahid, M. J., Alami, S. Y., Nassar, V. H., Balikian, J. B., and Salem, A. A.: Primary intestinal lymphoma with paraproteinemia. *Cancer 35:* 848–858, 1975.

47. Sherrick, D. W., Hodgson, J. R., and Dockerty, M. B.: The roentgenologic diagnosis of primary gastric lymphoma. *Radiology 84:* 925–932, 1965.

48. Smith, J. L., and Helwig, E. B.: Malignant lymphoma of the stomach; its diagnosis, distinction, and biologic behavior (abstract). *Am. J. Pathol. 34:* 553, 1958.

49. Stobbe, J. A., Dockerty, M. B., and Bernatz, P. E.: Primary gastric lymphoma and its grades

of malignancy. *Am. J. Surg. 112:* 10–19, 1966.

50. Thorbjarnarson, B., Beal, J. M., and Pearce, J. M.: Primary malignant lymphoid tumors of the stomach. *Cancer 9:* 712–717, 1956.
51. Thorbjarnarson, B., Pearce, J. M., and Beal, J. M.: Sarcoma of the stomach. *Am. J. Surg. 97:* 36–42, 1959.
52. Valdés-Dapena, A., Affolter, H., and Vilardell, F.: The gradient of malignancy in lymphoid lesions of the stomach. *Gastroenterology 50:* 382–389, 1966.
53. Warren, K. W.: Malignant lymphoma of the duodenum, small intestine and colon. *Surg. Clin. North Am. 39:* 725–735, 1959.
54. Warren, K. W., and Littlefield, J. B.: Malignant lymphomas of the gastrointestinal tract. *Surg. Clin. North Am. 35:* 735–746, 1955.
55. Warren, S., and Lulenski, C. R.: Primary solitary lymphoid tumors of the gastro-intestinal tract. *Ann. Surg. 115:* 1–12, 1942.
56. Wheelock, M. C., Atkinson, A. J., and Pizzo, A.: Lymphosarcoma of ileum. *Gastroenterology 15:* 158–161, 1950.
57. Wolf, B. S., and Marshall, R. H.: Roentgen features of diffuse lymphosarcoma of the colon. *Radiology 75:* 733–740, 1960.
58. Wolferth, C. C., Brady, L. W., Enterline, H. T., and Blakemore, W. S.: Primary lymphosarcoma of the stomach. *Surg. Gynecol. Obstet. 109:* 755–761, 1959.
59. Wychulis, A. R., Beahrs, O. H., and Woolner, L. B.: Malignant lymphoma of the colon; a study of 69 cases. *Arch. Surg. 93:* 215–225, 1966.
60. Yamashiro, K. M., and Gray, G. M.: Primary intestinal lymphoma; response to radiotherapy (abstract). *Clin. Res. 20:* 183, 1972.

Chapter 14

The Apudomas; with Particular Reference to Those of Gastroenteropancreatic Origin*

A. G. E. PEARSE

The term APUDOMA was derived by Szijj, Csapó, Lászlo, and Kovács[27] from the acronym APUD (Amine content and/or Amine Precursor Uptake and Decarboxylation) and the suffix 'oma'. The acronym was used by Pearse[15, 16] to describe a series of endocrine or potentially endocrine cells whose apparent main function was the synthesis and secretion of a peptide hormone or hormones. The Greek termination is habitually, if incorrectly, used to signify 'tumor'. The word apudoma thus accidentally represents an example of that classical linguistic outrage, a Latin-Greek hybrid.

The APUD cell series currently contains some 35 to 40 independent cell types, the majority of which are responsible for the production of either amine or peptide hormones, in some cases of both. The series is divided into central and peripheral divisions and, because the accumulated weight of evidence indicates that all its constituent cells are derivatives either of neural, or of specialized ectoderm, both divisions are regarded as neuroendocrine. Potential or actual peptide hormone-producing tumors arising from the individual cells of the APUD series, or from their direct precursors whether or not the latter are presently identifiable, are therefore to be regarded as apudomas.

The word *neurocristoma* has been suggested as an alternative to apudoma.[1] It is yet another Latin-Greek hybrid, preferable to the correct term *neurolophoma,* because it is more euphonious. If we allow the term 'crest' to stand not only for the neural crest but also for the neural ridges, for the neural tube itself, and for such specialized ectodermal derivatives as the placodes, then neurocristoma correctly describes the embryologic derivative of the apudomas. That name, however, is to be considered preferable for the whole series of APUD cell-derived tumors because it carries with it the functional implication of their potential for the production of amine and peptide hormones. It thus compels an awareness of their endocrine nature, even in the case of 'silent' examples of the tumor, which numerically exceed the clinically active variety by a wide margin.

* The work which formed the basis for this review was carried out with the assistance of a grant (SP 1215) from the Cancer Campaign.

GASTROINTESTINAL AND PANCREATIC APUD CELLS

The cells whose precursors are responsible for the production of gastroentero-pancreatic (GEP) apudomas constitute the major portion of the peripheral neuroendocrine division of the APUD series.[18] They are described in terms of the original Wiesbaden classification and its Bologna successor.[7, 25] The full list is given in Table 1. Also shown, in the two right-hand columns, are the proven, presumptive, or possible products of each of the cell types. Peptides or amines in these last two categories appear in Table 1 in brackets.

From the table it can be seen that the normal products of the GEP APUD cells include 12 peptides and 4 amines. Hormones other than these have not yet been shown to be produced by the 18 cells listed, but it is probable that with more refined and sensitive assay techniques other peptides will be found to be secreted in subphysiologic amounts.

THE APUDOMAS

The term apudoma requires two definitions, one biologic, the other patho-logic. Biologically an apudoma is a tumor, derived from an APUD cell and thus neuroectodermal in quality, which is secreting either its normal peptide hor-mone (or a variant thereof), or one or more of the hormones, prohormones, or carrier peptides of the APUD cell series, or, additionally or solely, one or more of the amine hormones associated with the series.

In pathologic terms, on the other hand, an apudoma is an "endocrine" tumor

TABLE 1. GASTROENTEROPANCREATIC APUD CELLS*

Cell*		Peptide	Amine
Stomach	G	Gastrin	—
	A or A-L	Pancreatic glucagon	—§
	EC$_1$	Substance P	5-HT
	ECL	—	(H)
	D	SRIF	—
Intestine	EC$_{1, 2}$	Motilin, Substance P	5-HT (MT)
	EG	Enteroglucagon	—
	S	Secretin	—
	D	SRIF	—
	D$_1$	(VIP)	—
	I	CCK	—
	K	GIP	—
	H	—	—
Pancreas	B	Insulin	DA, 5-HT†
	A	Glucagon	DA, 5-HT†
	D	SRIF	—
	D$_1$	VIP	—
	F	PP‡	—

* Letters indicate Wiesbaden classification, modified at Bologna 1973 (see Ref. 25). A-L, A-like; EC, enterochromaffin; 5-HT, 5-Hydroxytryptamine; ECL, EC-like; H, histamine; SRIF, somatostatin; CCK, cholecystokinin-pancreozymin; GIP, gastric inhibitory peptide; VIP, vasoactive intestinal peptide; MT, melatonin; DA, dopamine; PP, pancreatic peptide.

† Not in man; variable according to species.

‡ Usually prefixed by symbol H, B, or A to denote human, bovine, or avian origin.

§ Absent in most species.

possessing the amine-handling and associated cytochemical qualities of its presumptive precursor cell, characterized ultrastructurally by the presence of specific storage granules of endocrine type, containing a peptide component with or without a catechol or indolalkylamine. The peptide may or may not be identifiable by immunocytochemistry, and the amine may or may not be identifiable by cytofluorometry.

Apudomas are best described by the name of the principal peptide hormone which they are producing, if one can be identified, *e.g.*, insulinoma, gastrinoma. If the resulting word offends the ear the tumor can be described as an apudoma secreting, for example, cholecystokinin or 5-hydroxytryptamine. In the case of multiple peptide, or multiple peptide and amine production, use of the second type of nomenclature is obligatory.

The great majority of GEP apudomas fall into the class of carcinoid or carcinoid-islet tumors and of the remainder a substantial proportion can be classified as carcinomas. It is scarcely necessary, therefore, to illustrate the multiplicity of morphologic types by which the apudomas are represented. The diagnosis is made, entirely without bias from light microscopic morphology, by the use of cytochemical and ultrastructural criteria assisted by two or three simple histologic techniques. The various methods employed are given in Table 2.

The prime requirement for successful demonstration of any of the characteristics listed in Table 2 is appropriate preparation. In most cases this is synonymous with fixation and the type of fixation best employed can conveniently be considered for each section of Table 2 individually. It is unfortunate that, at present, no single method has been found which permits optimal expression of each of the light microscopic characteristics, while the ultrastructural ones have a complete requirement for glutaraldehyde-osmium tetroxide fixation. Nevertheless, even when the preparation of a particular tumor has been suboptimal, or worse, it is worthwhile to apply some of the simpler techniques in the list. Immunocytochemical methods, for instance, may still be able to identify hormones whose antibody-reacting sequences are relatively stable to the common fixatives.

HISTOLOGIC TECHNIQUES

The lead hematoxylin technique was adapted for studies of endocrine cells by Solcia, Capella and Vassallo.[24] It can be applied after many different fixatives,

TABLE 2. DIAGNOSTIC METHODS FOR APUDOMAS

Histologic techniques	Lead hematoxylin
	Masked metachromasia
	Argyrophilia
Nonspecific cytochemistry	α-Glycerophosphate dehydrogenase
	Esterases
	Cholinesterases
Specific cytochemistry	Formaldehyde-induced fluorescence (FIF)
	Uptake and decarboxylation of amine precursors (APUD-FIF)
Immunocytochemistry	Immunofluorescence
	Immunoperoxidase techniques
Ultrastructural microscopy	Endocrine granule analysis

including simple buffered formalin, and it demonstrates, with a considerable degree of reliability, the presence or absence of endocrine-type granules (Fig. 1). If the latter are absent it follows that those techniques listed in Table 1, which depend on the presence of a stored peptide or amine, will be unlikely to give positive results either.

The masked metachromasia method, also adapted by Solcia, Vassallo, and Capella[26] for endocrine cell studies, is best applied after fixation for 24 hours in 6% buffered glutaraldehyde, in Bouin's fluid, or in a glutaraldehyde-picric acid mixture. It is less useful than the other two methods in this section but has been shown by Rost and Rost,[23] in the case of the thyroid C cell granules, to depend wholly on their constituent peptides, and not on lipids or lipoproteins in the granule membrane or matrix. It can thus properly be considered as a cytochemical reaction.

Of the many silver staining techniques available the two most reliable are, for argentaffinity, the Masson-Fontana method, and for argyrophilia, the method of Grimelius.[10] The first of these gives a positive result only if the granules contain an amine whose formaldehyde condensation product is capable of reducing alkaline silver solutions directly. The second gives a positive result with the granules of the vast majority of endocrine tumors though it has a threshold

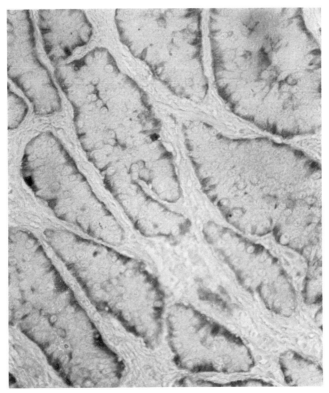

FIG. 1. "Carcinoid" tumor removed from the kidney of a female aged 45. Lead hematoxylin technique after fixation in buffered formalin at pH 7.2. Shows basal granular content of the tumor cells later shown by immunocytochemistry to cross-react with antisera to pancreatic glucagon. × 150.

above the level reached by electron microscopy where, theoretically at least, a single endocrine granule per section is detectable.

NONSPECIFIC CYTOCHEMISTRY.

The three enzymes for which methods are described in this section are by no means uniformly strongly reactive in all the APUD cells of the GEP system.[17] They are, on the other hand, invariably so in tumors arising from the cells of the series. Fresh frozen cryostat sections are required for the demonstration of α-glycerophosphate dehydrogenase (Fig. 2) while overnight fixation in methanol-free formaldehyde is best for the two esterases.[22]

SPECIFIC CYTOCHEMISTRY

Formaldehyde-induced fluorescence (FIF) is studied in tissues quenched in Freon 12 or 22 at $-158°$ and subsequently freeze-dried and fixed with formaldehyde vapor at 60 to 80° for 1 to 3 hours.[8] Uptake of the amine precursors 5-hydroxytryptophan and 3,4-dihydroxyphenylalanine (A-P-U-D) is conveniently investigated by the *in vitro* method of Häkanson, Lilja, and Owman,[11] followed by the FIF procedure.

IMMUNOCYTOCHEMISTRY

A number of alternative preparative techniques have been described in the literature for the preservation of peptide antigens. Of the routine fixatives one of

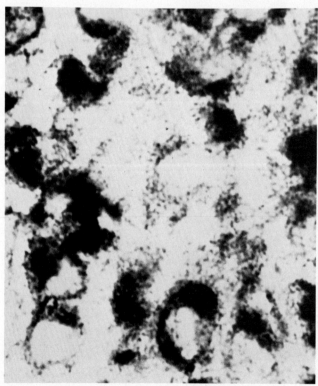

FIG. 2. "Amelanotic melanoma" in male aged 56. The tumor cells contain extremely high levels of menadione-linked α-glycerophosphate dehydrogenase. $\times$ 920.

the best is Bouin's fluid and many hormones are adequately preserved by buffered and, especially, methanol-free formaldehyde (3 to 4 hours at 4°). For certain labile peptides improved preservation may be obtained by the use of 10% carbodiimide in phosphate buffer[13] or by using diethylpyrocarbonate applied as a vapor (at 55° for 3 hours) to freeze-dried blocks.[20] From a large number of bifunctional reagents tested as liquid fixatives for hormone peptides dimethyl-suberimidate[12] and *p*-benzoquinone[19] were found superior to all others. Variations of the direct and indirect immunofluorescence techniques of Coons, Leduc, and Connolly[3] and of the immunoperoxidase technique of Nakane and Pierce[14] are employed, to some extent, according to the personal preference of the operator. Gastrin immunofluorescence in some of the cells of a small carcinoid, from the wall of the duodenum in a male aged 82, is illustrated in Figure 3. In this formalin-fixed preparation no other peptide could be demonstrated in the gastrin-negative cells. Negative results are of no significance in immunocyto-chemical practice, however. The most important need is for antisera of known specificity and high avidity. Commercial antisera are available for a number of peptide hormones. They vary widely in quality, as do those sera which are produced privately.

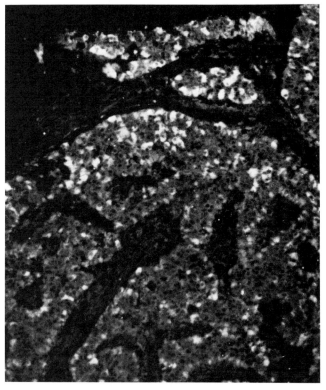

FIG. 3. "Carcinoid" tumor. Autopsy finding in male aged 82. Indirect immunofluorescence with antigastrin serum shows cross-reactivity with the protein stored in endocrine type granules. The diagnosis was, therefore, silent gastrinoma. × 94.

ULTRASTRUCTURAL MICROSCOPY

Conventional techniques for ultrastructural morphology are applied to endocrine peptide tumors essentially for a single reason. This is to establish the presence or absence in the tumor cells of "endocrine" granules and, if possible, to make some sort of identification of the nature of their contained hormones, both amine and peptide.

The identification of normal GEP cells by electron microscopy can be undertaken with confidence, and here, once established, the identity of the product of any given cell type is thereafter assumed. In Figure 4 are shown, in the human fundus, parts of a parietal cell, a (D) cell, and an EC-like (ECL) cell. The D cell was assumed, and is now proven, to be producing somatostatin, and the product of the ECL cell is still unknown. The identification of the peptide product in an

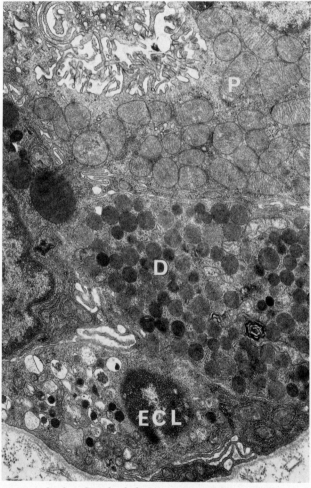

FIG. 4. Human gastric fundus. Standard electron microscopic preparation counterstained with uranyl acetate and lead citrate. Below the parietal cell (*P*) are parts of two endocrine cells. The first is a *D* cell (somatostatin), the other an EC-like (ECL) cell. × 12,500.

apudoma, from the nature of its contained granules, is far more difficult, and usually impossible.

DIAGNOSIS OF GEP APUDOMAS: FURTHER CONSIDERATIONS

It must be made clear that once a tumor of the gastroenteropancreatic system has been diagnosed, even tentatively, by light microscopic histology and cyto-chemistry as an apudoma, pride of place has to be given to the methods of immunocytochemistry and electron microscopy. An absolute (but not necessarily complete) diagnosis can be made if a positive result is obtained with a specific peptide antiserum. If electron microscopy reveals granules of endocrine type these may or may not confirm clinically based indications of the hormonal nature of the tumor, and any immunocytochemical or serum radioimmuno- and biologic assays which may have been made.

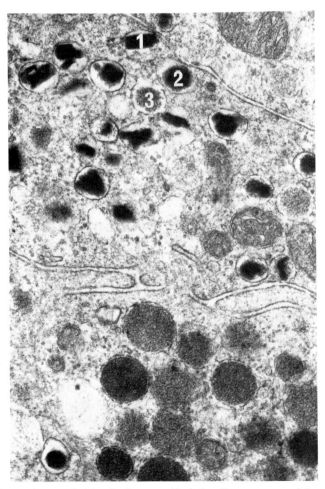

FIG. 5. Electron micrograph (standard preparation). Insulinoma removed from pancreas of a female aged 42. Shown above: 1) classical paracrystalline B granules, 2) classical non-crystalline electron dense B granules with halo, 3) fine granular B granules. Below, right, part of a D cell, associated with a single B granule. × 30,000.

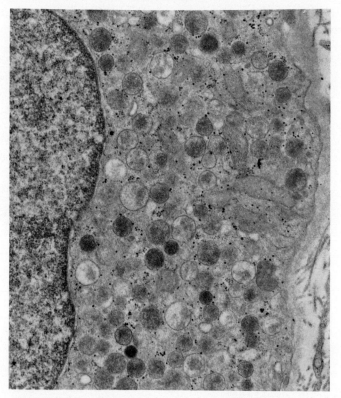

Fɪɢ. 6. Electron micrograph (standard preparation). Shows part of a classical gastrin (G) cell from human antrum. This appearance is seldom seen in pancreatic or extrapancreatic gastrinomas. × 18,000.

Iɴsᴜʟɪɴᴏᴍᴀs

Creutzfeldt and coworkers[5] made a very thorough analysis of the functional status and morphology of a series of 30 insulinomas. In associated studies Creutzfeldt *et al.*,[5] indicated that the principal metabolic failure of neoplastic B cells was a failure of storage, and their morphologic data confirmed the frequent low level of granularity in the tumor cells. Although it is possible to show non-granule-bound insulin if a sufficient quantity is present it is usually impossible to demonstrate insulin or any other hormone in tumor cells shown by electron microscopy to be free of granules.

If the classical human B granules, in their paracystalline form, are present (Fig. 5) absolute identification of an insulinoma can be made without recourse to immunocytochemistry. This is one of the very few cases where an ultrastructural identification can be made with such confidence. A second type of granule, illustrated in Figure 1, can also be diagnosed as insulin-containing. This is the dense core granule with the large clear halo. A third type of granule, with a small halo and finely granular content or lower electron density, is commonly regarded as containing proinsulin but no acceptable proof of this view has been given.

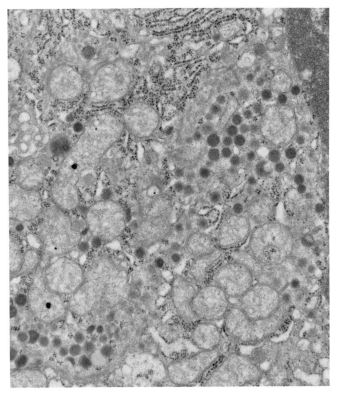

Fig. 7. Pancreatic gastrinoma, standard electron microscopic preparation. Shows atypical small, round, moderately osmiophilic granules (mean diameter, 165 nm). These cannot be equated with the granules of any known gastroenteropancreatic (GEP) endocrine cell. × 18,000.

Gastrinomas

The diagnosis of gastrinomas (non-G cell gastrin-producing tumors) of the pancreas was considered by Vassallo, Solcia, Bussolati, Polak, and Pearse,[28] who concluded that the then available evidence supported the view that pancreatic gastrinomas arose from the D cell, at that time (erroneously) considered to be the source of pancreatic gastrin.[9] In a more recent review of their work Creutzfeldt, Arnold, Creutzfeldt, and Track[6] indicated that in 9 of their 10 gastrinomas the Grimelius silver reaction was positive. They divided their tumors, ultrastructurally, into four types. Type I, containing typical G-cell granules (Fig. 6), permitted ultrastructural diagnosis of gastrinoma to be made, as did their type II with a mixture of typical and atypical G-cell granules. Type III tumors contained only atypical granules (Fig. 7) but these, as shown in Figure 8, are reliably demonstrated as argyrophil by the Grimelius silver technique. The last Type (IV) was represented by a single case containing endocrine cells of several different types. The authors drew attention to the presence, in their pancreatic gastrinomas, of cells containing other (normal) hormones, particularly insulin, and this has been reemphasized in a new appraisal of the whole problem of the origin of pancreatic endocrine tumors by Creutzfeldt.[4]

Multihormone Tumors

The problem of multihormone tumors is a difficult one. Even when two or more hormone products have been identified in a tumor, by extraction and radioimmunoassay, or by immunocytochemistry, it may be difficult or even impossible to determine whether they are products of a single cell type or not. Most published cases of multihormone tumors report the presence of distinct cell types of each hormone. The position was well summed up by Bordi and Bussolati,[2] who found that 3 out of their 4 multihormone pancreatic apudomas contained more than one endocrine cell type. More recently Polak, Bloom, Adrian, Heitz, Bryant, and Pearse[21] found pancreatic polypeptide in more than half of 33 pancreatic apudomas, and in their hepatic and lymph node metastases when these were available. The tumors were primarily insulinomas, gastrinomas, glucagonomas, and vipomas, all of which had been considered originally to be producing a single hormone. Pancreatic polypeptide was not found in GEP tumors of nonpancreatic origin and the reason for its production by such a high proportion of pancreatic apudomas remains to be elucidated.

Other GEP Apudomas

In addition to the two principle gastroenteropancreatic peptide-producing apudomas (insulinoma, gastrinoma) there are recorded accounts of the identifi-

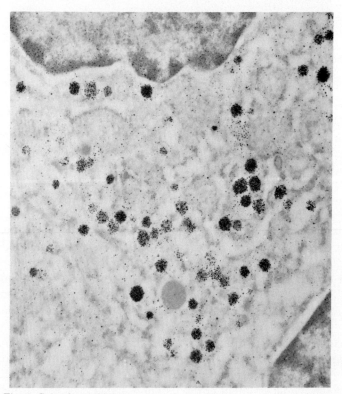

Fig. 8. As Fig. 7. Grimelius silver preparation. Shows strong to moderate argyrophilia in the atypical granules of this gastrinoma. × 18,000.

cation of several others. Glucagonomas, vipomas, and a single example of each enteroglucagonoma and gipoma have been described. Authentic, assay-proven, examples of secretinoma and cholecystokininoma are not yet available. Somatostatinomas, motilinomas, and Substance P'omas surely cannot fail to exist. We can only await their revelation, along with many other factual recordings which may ultimately enable us to solve not only Creutzfeldt's riddle of the origin of pancreatic endocrine tumors, but the enigma of all the apudomas of the gastroenteropancreatic system.

REFERENCES

1. Bolande, R. P.: The neurocristopathies; a unifying concept of disease arising in neural crest maldevelopment. *Hum. Pathol. 5:* 409–429, 1974.
2. Bordi, C., and Bussolati, G.: Immunofluorescence, histochemical and ultrastructural studies for the detection of multiple endocrine polypeptide tumours of the pancreas. *Virchows Archiv. (Cell Pathol.) 17:* 13–27, 1974.
3. Coons, A. H., Leduc, E. H., and Connolly, J. M.: Studies on antibody production. I. A method for the histochemical demonstration of specific antibody and its application to a study of the hyperimmune rabbit. *J. Exp. Med. 102:* 49–60, 1955.
4. Creutzfeldt, W.: Pancreatic endocrine tumors—the riddle of their origin and hormone secretion. *Isr. J. Med. Sci. 11:* 762–776, 1975.
5. Creutzfeldt, W., Arnold, R., Creutzfeldt, C., Deuticke, U., Frerichs, H., and Track, N. S.: Biochemical and morphological investigations of 30 human insulinomas. Correlation between the tumour content of insulin and proinsulin-like components and the histological and ultrastructural appearance. *Diabetologia 9:* 217–231, 1973.
6. Creutzfeldt, W., Arnold, R., Creutzfeldt, C., and Track, N. S.: Pathomorphologic, biochemical and diagnositc aspects of gastrinomas (Zollinger-Ellison syndrome). *Hum. Pathol. 6:* 47–76, 1975.
7. Creutzfeldt, W., Gregory, R. A., Grossman, M. I., and Pearse, A. G. E. (eds.): *Origin, chemistry, physiology and pathophysiology of the gastrointestinal hormones.* Proceedings of the International Symposium at Wiesbaden, 1969, p. 95. Stuttgart, F. K. Schattauer-Verlag, 1970.
8. Falck, B., and Owman, C.: A detailed methodological description of the fluorescence method for the cellular demonstration of biogenic monoamines. *Acta Univ. Lund (Section II):* No. 7, 1–23, 1965.
9. Greider, M H., and McGuigan, J. E.: Cellular localization of gastrin in the human pancreas. *Diabetes 20:* 389–396, 1971.
10. Grimelius, L.: A silver nitrate stain for α_2 cells in human pancreatic islets. *Acta Soc. Med. Upsal. 73:* 243–270, 1968.
11. Häkanson, R., Lilja, B., and Owman, Ch.: Properties of a new system of amine-storing cells in the gastric mucosa of the rat. *Eur. J. Pharmacol. 1:* 188–199, 1967.
12. Hassell, J., and Hand, A. R.: Tissue fixation with diimidoesters as an alternative to aldehydes. I. Comparison of cross-linking and ultrastructure obtained with dimethylsuberimidate and glutaraldehyde. *J. Histochem. Cytochem. 22:* 223–239, 1974.
13. Kendall, P. A., Polak, J. M., and Pearse, A. G. E.: Carbodiimide fixation for immunohistochemistry; observations on the fixation of polypeptide hormones. *Experientia 27:* 1104–1106, 1971.
14. Nakane, P. K., and Pierce, G. B., Jr.: Enzyme-labeled antibodies for the light and electron macroscopic localization of tissue antigens. *J. Cell Biol. 33:* 307–318, 1967.
15. Pearse, A. G. E.: Common cytochemical and ultrastructural characteristics of cells producing polypeptide hormones (the APUD series) and their relevance to thyroid and ultimobranchial C cells and calcitonin. *Proc. R. Soc. Lond. (Biol.) 170:* 71–80, 1968.
16. Pearse, A. G. E.: The cytochemistry and ultrastructure of polypeptide hormone-producing cells of the APUD series and the embryologic, physiologic and pathologic implications of the concept. *J. Histochem. Cytochem. 17:* 303–313, 1969.
17. Pearse, A. G. E.: *Histochemistry, Theoretical and Applied,* 3rd ed., vol. 2, Edinburgh and

London, Churchill Livingstone, 1972.

18. Pearse, A. G. E.: Neurocristopathy, neuroendocrine pathology and the APUD concept. *Z. Krebsforsch. 84:* 1–18, 1975.

19. Pearse, A. G. E., and Polak, J. M.: Bifunctional reagents as vapour-and liquid-phase fixatives for immunohistochemistry. *Histochem. J. 7:* 179–186, 1975.

20. Pearse, A. G. E., Polak, J. M., Adams, C., and Kendall, P. A.: Diethylpyrocarbonate, a vapour-phase fixative for immunofluorescence studies on polypeptide hormones. *Histochem. J. 6:* 347–352, 1974.

21. Polak, J. M., Bloom, S. R., Adrian, T. E., Heitz, Ph., Bryant, M. G., and Pearse, A. G. E.: Pancreatic polypeptide in insulinomas, gastrinomas, vipomas and glucagonomas. *Lancet 1:* 328–330, 1976.

22. Polak, J. M., Bussolati, G., and Pearse, A. G. E.: Cytochemical, immunofluorescence and ultrastructural investigations on the antral G cells in hyperparathyroidism. *Virchows Archiv. (Cell Pathol.) 9:* 187–197, 1971.

23. Rost, M. C. M., and Rost, F. W. D.: Storage granules of thyroid C cells in the dog; a cytochemical and ultrastructural study, in relation to the masked metachromasia reaction. *Histochem. J. 7:* 307–320, 1975.

24. Solcia, E., Capella, C., Vassallo, G.: Lead haematoxylin as a stain for endocrine cells; significance of staining and comparison with other selective methods. *Histochemie 20:* 116–126, 1969.

25. Solcia, E., Pearse, A. G. E., Grube, D., Kobayashi, S., Bussolati, G., Creutzfeldt, W., and Gepts, W.: Revised Wiesbaden classification of gut endocrine cells. *Rendic. Gastroenterol. 5:* 13–16, 1973.

26. Solcia, E., Vassallo, G., and Capella, C.: Selective staining of endocrine cells by basic dyes after acid hydrolysis. *Stain Technol. 43:* 257–263, 1968.

27. Szijj, J. I., Csapó, Z., Lászlo, F. A., and Kovács, K.: Medullary cancer of the thyroid gland associated with hypercorticism. *Cancer 24:* 167–173, 1969.

28. Vassallo, G., Solcia, E., Bussolati, G., Polak, J. M., and Pearse, A. G. E.: Non-G cell gastrin-producing tumours of the pancreas. *Virchows Archiv. (Cell Pathol.) 11:* 66–79, 1972.

Index

Page references in *italic* type refer to illustrations.